Truth, Lies and the OR

The Good, the Bad and the Realities

By

F. W. Ernst, M.D.
William G. Pace III, M. D.

In collaboration with
Dinah Blankenship
and
Tom Nugent

Warren Publishing, Inc.

F. W. Ernst, M.D. — William G. Pace III, M. D.

Disclaimer: This book contains true case histories. In order to preserve the privacy of the people involved, we have made changes in locales, names, and certain aspects of the personal stories so they are not identifiable. Any resemblance to any persons, living or dead, is strictly coincidental.

Copyright © 2008
Frederick W. Ernst, M. D.

All rights reserved. No part of this publication may be reproduced, stored in a retrieval system, or transmitted in any form or any other means electronic, mechanical, photocopying, recording or otherwise, without the prior written permission of the publisher.

Published by Warren Publishing, Inc.
www.warrenpublishing.net

ISBN: 1-886057-59-1

Printed in the United States of America

(Parts of this text have been previously published under the title: *Now They Lay Me Down to Sleep*)

This book is dedicated to the memory of

William G. Pace, III, M.D.

He was my teacher, a patient advocate extraordinaire, my esteemed co-author, and my very dear friend.

TABLE OF CONTENTS

Foreword..i

Acknowledgments..iii

Chapter 1   Hospital Admission..1

Chapter 2   Selecting your Surgeon......................................13

Chapter 3   Anesthesia Care Providers—
            "Who will watch over me while I sleep?"................29

Chapter 4   Preparing Children—
            "I am not a small adult."..43

Chapter 5   Beauty for a Fatal Price......................................53

Chapter 6   Foreign Medical Graduates................................67

Chapter 7   Doc In A Box...77

Chapter 8   Office-Based Surgery...91

Chapter 9   Awareness under General Anesthesia..............119

Chapter 10 To Sue or Not to Sue..135

Chapter 11 Malpractice Options...153

Chapter 12 Lessons for Everyone.......................................171

Epilogue..189

Afterword...193

About the Authors..197

About the Editors...199

Glossary...201

FOREWORD

In the years since our first medical consumer advocacy book **Now They Lay Me Down To Sleep** came off the press, I have been privileged to see the book in the hands of over eight thousand Americans and to speak to thousands more in large and small groups and on local and national television and radio. The book's purpose was to help people—you, the consumer of medical services and products—understand how to make wiser choices in selecting health care providers.

The response to this book has been overwhelmingly positive, including affirmative feedback from others in the medical profession. Publication in 1996 launched my second career as a patients' rights advocate. Speaking to groups nationwide on current medical consumer issues now involves much of my time. In the intervening years since **Now They Lay Me Down To Sleep** appeared, two areas of medicine have exploded: *office-based surgery* and *awareness under general anesthesia.*

Twenty-five percent of all surgery today in America is done in the office setting. Unfortunately, major disasters and/or complications continue to happen in the office setting even in states with guidelines designed to prevent this. My medical-legal expert witness work further validates this unfortunate fact.

Twenty-eight states lack any office surgery guidelines; of the 22 states with guidelines, a number of them have regulations that are insufficient to ensure safety and quality of care. Over 75 percent of my speaking engagements are in the states with no guidelines or insufficient ones.

Awareness under general anesthesia has been receiving increased media coverage. In this procedure, a patient is not fully anesthetized to the point that he or she is oblivious to the operating room situation. The patient can hear conversation and may feel pain, something he or she

F. W. Ernst, M.D. — William G. Pace III, M. D.

cannot communicate because muscle relaxants used as part of the anesthesia temporarily cause paralysis. Many patients have described this phenomenon as a "horrendous, nightmarish experience," leaving them with residual anger towards the anesthesia profession, apprehensive about future anesthesia, and problems with post traumatic stress syndrome.

In view of these two growing medical issues—office-based surgery and awareness under general anesthesia—I felt it was time to publish a new updated medical consumer advocacy book with two new chapters devoted to these topics.

Although the American public has come a long way toward becoming more knowledgeable and proactive medical consumers, we still have much to achieve. I believe greater knowledge and understanding of medical practices, combined with individual proactivity as medical consumers, will lead us to higher standards of care, higher rates of successful treatment, and decreased instances of medical malpractice suits.

Working together, we can create for ourselves and others a stronger and safer American health care system.

Frederick W. Ernst, M.D.
March 1, 2008

ACKNOWLEDGMENTS

An undertaking such as this book could not be accomplished without the help and moral support of many people. This project has truly been a team effort.

To my wife, Maureen, I offer loving thanks for your understanding, patience, and encouragement over these past months of work on the book.

To Cathy Brophy, President of Warren Publishing, who has been my personal editor at Warren, I extend my heartfelt thanks and gratitude. She said from the start, "I want to do this project myself." I could not have asked for a better editor or more superlative results.

To Dinah Blankenship, Tom Nugent, and Dr. Nancy G. Spear, I extend kudos to you for your valuable contributions. They took all our original writings in various forms and developed them into the final draft that was submitted to Warren Publishing.

To Sydni Ann Shollenberger and Robert Fitzgerald, my personal literary advisers, I hope you are pleased with the end result. Many thanks.

To Dr. Paul Howard who offered expert advice and guidance on the revision of Chapter 5, thank you so much.

To our endorsers who believed in our commitment to patients' rights, I extend our sincere thanks.

Throughout the writing of this book, I have felt the gentle spirit of my co-author, Bill Pace, guiding me along every step of the way. Bill, I hope you are proud of the final product.

Finally, there are many others who have helped along the way. You know that I value the support and services of every single one of you. If, together, you and we have helped save families from anguish and needless tragedies, we have accomplished our mission.

F. W. Ernst, M.D. — William G. Pace III, M. D.

Truth, Lies and the OR

CHAPTER ONE

HOSPITAL ADMISSION

Dr. Spear

KEY POINTS:

- **Warning to Surgical/Anesthesia Patients: Admission Is Not A "Routine Procedure!"**
- **Choosing the Right Hospital for Surgery is a Vital Part of Obtaining Quality Care.**

QUESTION: How important is it to select the right hospital?
ANSWER: Crucial.
Why? Listen to the hair-raising story of 70-year-old Fred Chambers of North Carolina, who landed in a medical facility that failed miserably to fulfill its stated mission "to provide the very best medical care for each patient's special needs"...

****

Little Bobby's birthday party was going to be glorious. Fred Chambers had seen to that. A retired printer living in Charlotte, North Carolina, Fred had been looking forward to his grandson's birthday for several weeks now. And why not? Living comfortably on his Social Security and monthly pension check from Allied Print Products, the fun-loving Chambers had plenty of time to spend on his seven grandkids. And little Bobby, a freckled third-grader with a passion for cheeseburgers, was his absolute favorite.

F. W. Ernst, M.D. — William G. Pace III, M. D.

Still young at heart, Chambers had rented a small birthday room at the neighborhood Kangaroo Kids Restaurant out on Greenspring Avenue. He had bought at least 400 balloons and some of the goofiest-looking party hats in the history of kiddiedom. Then, with generous good spirit still flowing, he urged Bobby's mom—his daughter Claire—to invite a dozen or so of the boy's schoolmates to the festive affair.

So far, so good. By five o'clock on that Saturday afternoon in April 1997, the blowout at the Kangaroo Kids place was in full blast, with a dozen youngsters furiously gobbling cake and ice cream, hurling party streamers, singing endless renditions of the "Road Runner" song, and, in general, behaving like rambunctious kids without a worry in the world.

Fred Chambers was having the time of his life.

A prank-playing rascal who loved to spend hours with his grandchildren, the light-hearted Chambers zipped around the birthday party in high style. He helped several youngsters blow up balloons and then assisted his grandson to pin the tail on a particularly elusive donkey.

Around six o'clock the trouble began.

All at once, as he batted a "Spiderman" balloon toward a couple of Bobby's classmates, Fred Chambers began to feel woozy, light-headed.

He sat down hard on one of the plastic folding chairs that Kangaroo Kids had provided for the party. His shoulders slumped, and he began to shake his head back and forth in a futile effort to "get rid of the cobwebs."

But nothing helped. With each passing minute, he grew weaker, dizzier . . . until suddenly Claire was at his side.

"Dad . . . what is it? You're white as a sheet!"

Truth, Lies and the OR

With horror, Claire then watched her father slide from his chair and topple face-first onto the carpeted floor!

Within seconds, the ambulance had been summoned, and the sirens were shrieking outside the door of the restaurant.

Claire rode with him to the emergency room at Carstairs General Hospital, located on the southern outskirts of Charlotte.

As they raced into the emergency room, the attendants were already succeeding in bringing the retired printer back to consciousness.

Claire hung onto his hand. "Can you hear me, Dad? Can you move your hand?"

She held her breath . . . then nearly burst into tears when his eyes fluttered open, and he actually managed to joke, "Maybe I ate too many french fries!"

In a flash, the ER-crew was hard at work. After stabilizing his vital signs and determining that there was no immediate threat to the patient's life, the medical technicians began running a series of tests aimed at uncovering the cause of the collapse.

Because their medical assessment showed that there had been no "residual neurological deficit," the attending physician noted the probable cause of the fainting as a small stroke or perhaps a heart blockage. And that was it: with the patient sitting up now and cracking jokes, apparently normal, he was bundled up and then admitted to a floor for observation.

Incredibly enough, however, the hospital personnel who took Fred Chambers through the admitting process were about to commit one of the cardinal sins of placing a patient in a ward.

For reasons that to this day remain unclear, the staff at Carstairs General took no measures to provide nursing care, restraints, or bedside rails—elements of good patient management that clearly were mandated in the case of a 70-year-old man who had already collapsed once earlier that day.

Nor did the hospital authorities think it necessary to alert Fred Chambers' family to the possibility that he might need special attention from family members, to prevent the possibility of a dangerous fall from his hospital bed.

Once this unfortunate scenario had been put in place, the results were virtually inevitable.

First, Mr. Chambers was sedated. Then he was put on bed rest, without restraints. As anyone might have predicted, he responded to this regimen the way any layman might: awakening early the next morning, he attempted to climb out of bed in order to visit the bathroom.

He fell hard.

When the nurses found him a few minutes later, he was crawling along the floor of the ward, shaken but apparently uninjured. He was quickly examined, and the X-rays showed no evidence of a hip fracture or other deformity (a typical outcome, in such falls by elderly patients).

With no broken bones or lesions showing in the radiologic exam, the patient was returned to his floor.

Within four or five days, however, he gradually became unable to stand on his left leg, due to severe pain in his left hip. But the treatment he received next only made matters worse.

An astute clinician would have immediately re-examined the hip. He or she would also have remembered a key medical danger always present in this situation: the possibility that an "impacted subcapital fracture" might not show up on X-ray, but might instead persist for several days until, with the collapse of nearby tissue, the bone actually separated and the fracture became clinically apparent.

Truth, Lies and the OR

Unhappily, that's exactly the scenario that unfolded in the case of Fred Chambers.

During the next few weeks, the patient developed an obvious deformity of the left hip and was taken to the operating room, where a "resection" of the head of the femur and an artificial replacement were carried out. But it was too little, too late: by the time of this major surgery, the patient was deteriorating badly and had already declined into "serious" condition.

Tragically—and almost unbelievably—Fred Chambers never did recover from the surgery on his hip.

Although one could argue medically that, because of his age, Fred Chambers would probably have experienced some difficulty after such a fall—even with prompt, effective medical attention—there is little doubt that the hospital's mismanagement of his case contributed significantly to his untimely death, only four months after his admission to the hospital.

Claire Hargrove, Fred Chambers' daughter, collected a hefty malpractice settlement in this case a few years later. She now lives, however, with the knowledge that the primary cause of her father's early death was mismanagement of the hospital admitting process.

With proper admission procedures, calling for either bed restraints or nursing care, he would not have fallen from bed.

If he had received a complete physical exam and evaluation at the time of the original injury, the fracture could have been treated immediately, thus improving the patient's chances for a good outcome.

That was not what happened, though, for Fred Chambers. We can, however, learn from this powerful example of the crucial importance of the hospital admission process, focusing careful attention on every aspect of effective patient care.

F. W. Ernst, M.D. — William G. Pace III, M. D.

****

Rx: Hospital admission before surgery: getting it right

After you agree to surgery—and I emphasize the word "agree," because it is ultimately your decision whether or not to opt for surgery and/or anesthesia—several different medical processes begin to unfold.

Some of the initial steps will be under your control, and some will not. One of the early factors you will not likely be able to control is your health insurance package, unless you are fortunate enough to have received a health care plan to cover all contingencies.

Your insurance will significantly affect the admission process and determine your allowable length of stay in the hospital and the extent of postoperative home care and rehabilitative services. Furthermore, your insurance will determine the amount of money your surgeon, hospital, and anesthesia care team receive for their services.

Those who belong to a HMO (Health Maintenance Organization) will quickly discover that HMO physicians are required to contact their organization's claims department in order to retrieve guidelines for your pending surgery and to obtain permission for payment, referred to as "prior approval."

If your HMO is footing the bill, another key item to remember is that, should your physical condition require the services of a specialist (e.g. cardiovascular, orthopedic, or plastic surgeon), you will be required to obtain permission from your primary care physician before you can even make an appointment to see a surgeon or specialist.

After the surgeon has examined you, performed necessary diagnostic studies, and obtained approval from the HMO or other insurance company to proceed, you must weigh your options and decide whether or not to have surgery.

Truth, Lies and the OR

If you are paying cash or have private insurance as opposed to a Health Maintenance Organization plan, you can complete your admission without special permission from anyone.

With the preadmission steps clearly in mind and your decision to proceed with surgery made, let's consider:

- What actually occurs in a hospital admission?
- Key strategies for getting through admission with minimal stress
- Ways to assure the best medical outcome for you during a hospital stay

The hospital admission process will be based on the level of care your surgical team anticipates you to need during your particular procedure.

There are four basic admitting categories available to the surgical team in most hospital settings:

1. If you are expected to undergo surgery, recover within a few hours, then return home for a complete recovery, you will be admitted to and discharged from a special unit or facility designed for rapid processing of surgery and anesthesia. This unit is commonly referred to as the "Ambulatory Care Center" or "short stay area."
2. If your surgeon has any special concerns regarding your postoperative well-being, or if you will require intravenous pain medication, antibiotics, or experience persistent nausea and/or vomiting, the medical professionals may decide to admit you to the hospital overnight, which is considered a 23-hour admission.
3. A direct hospital admission is accomplished by simply reporting to the Admissions Department of the hospital. New state-of-the-art technology will allow you to go straight to a

designated area where an admitting clerk will complete the process with a laptop computer at bedside. Laboratory technicians will be available to draw blood for chemical analysis, and an EKG (electrocardiogram) and/or X-rays may be ordered.
4. An "emergency admission" occurs when a patient is admitted directly to the hospital from the emergency room.

Another important consideration to include in setting up the best possible scenario for successful surgery and recovery is the testing beforehand. Particularly if you are having surgery as an outpatient and your age or medical condition warrants, you should undergo several basic laboratory tests to check the condition of your heart, lungs, kidneys, and blood prior to the date of surgery.

Patients over age 50 are generally required to have a pre-operative electrocardiogram (EKG) and a chest X-ray. Some ambulatory care centers will arrange a visit with an anesthesia department representative for a pre-operative interview before the actual surgery date; others require this visit on the day of surgery.

If your body mass index (BMI) is 35 or greater, you will probably be requested to meet with a member of the anesthesia department at least 48 hours prior to date of your surgery. This is deemed necessary because scientific data suggests that borderline morbid obesity patients have a higher incidence of undiagnosed co-existing medical conditions which may increase the risks of surgical and/or anesthetic complications. A review of your complete medical evaluation prior to arriving for surgery, in a non-threatening environment, will help to identify any unrecognized medical problems and have them treated properly to avoid cancellation on the day of surgery. You and your anesthesia provider can focus on your health-care problems and candidly discuss the risks and benefits of different anesthesia techniques.

In most cases, a member of the ambulatory care staff will phone you at home, prior to the day of your scheduled surgery. A registered nurse (RN) or other medical professional will ask you about your medical history and present state of health to determine whether you are in the best possible physical condition for the anticipated anesthesia and surgery.

Your responses will be evaluated by medical professionals and those responses that seem unusual, or significantly deviate from the norm, will require consultation with a member of the anesthesia department in order to decide whether additional diagnostic studies are needed.

Among the questions you should hear from your interview are:

- Do you have any drug or latex allergies?
- Are you currently taking medications? If so, what are they, in what dosages, and how often? If the list of medications is long or difficult to remember, take the medications with you to the hospital in the original bottles dispensed by the pharmacy.
- Do you have asthma or any other difficulties with breathing? Are you a smoker?
- Do you have hypertension, irregular heart beats, or other heart disease?
- Have you experienced seizures or a recent loss of memory?
- Do you have diabetes?
- Have you been treated for any major illnesses or infections within the past 6 months?

Your interviewer will also tell you which medications you may take on the morning of surgery and instruct you on eating and drinking restrictions prior to the surgical appointment.

F. W. Ernst, M.D. — William G. Pace III, M. D.

To prevent unnecessary delays or even cancellation of surgery, you must follow the pre-operative instructions. Some patients think that a few alcoholic beverages the night before surgery will make the surgery process less painful. Sorry! That's a losing strategy because, although a high blood alcohol level may temporarily lower your anxiety, it may also be the basis for declaring you incompetent to sign your consent for anesthesia and surgery, resulting in a postponement of your surgery.

Once you are admitted to the hospital and all necessary documents have been signed, you may request some pre-anesthetic medication (i.e. Versed) to help reduce your anxiety. If you have experienced post-op nausea and/or vomiting with past anesthetics, you can also request medications to reduce the possibility of a reoccurrence (i.e. Zofran, Pepcid, or a scopolamine patch).

So what should you expect when you check into a typical hospital?

On arrival, you'll meet someone in the reception area who will ask you various questions regarding your medical history. In teaching hospitals—often associated with universities—the number of people who greet you may be greater because teaching hospitals offer a larger number of health care providers. Your list of well-wishers and interviewers at admission could include nurses, nurses' aides, physicians' assistants, interns, residents, nurse anesthetists, anesthesiologists, your surgeon, and additional trainees from other hospital departments.

Be forewarned: you may be asked the same questions several times! Try not to become irritated at such repetitions. Through long experience, hospital staff members have learned that many patients—intimidated by unfamiliar surroundings and anxious about their well-being—forget important medical information and remember their complete medical histories only with repeated questioning. The inquiring process may reveal important facts about drug allergies, complications with specific anesthetic agents during previous surgeries, or physical injuries that could affect the choice of anesthetics, surgical procedures, and positioning on the OR table.

For many of us, the process of admission seems long, confusing, and repetitious. Still, you'll help yourself most as a patient if you remain calm and answer all questions honestly and clearly, all the while listening carefully to, and later abiding by, all instructions concerning your preoperative preparation. Although you will receive a set of written discharge instructions, having someone with you during the discharge process will aid you immensely in remembering and carrying out the discharge orders.

In 2000, the Institute of Medicine (IOM) released its report, "To Err Is Human—Building a Safer Health System." This report was the result of the IOM's federally-funded investigation into errors in American hospitals and put forth recommendations for improvement in quality of care and patient safety.

The report stated that as many as 100,000 Americans die a year in American hospitals as a result of preventable errors. This is greater than the number of deaths from motor vehicle accidents (43,458), breast cancer (43, 2009), or AIDS (16,516). The total national costs of preventable adverse events were estimated to be between $17 billion and $29 billion.

Generally speaking, American medical consumers believe that hospitals are a safe environment. In the eyes of the public, licensing and accreditation are synonymous with a "Good Housekeeping Seal of Approval." Yet, according to the IOM's report, licensing and accreditation processes have historically had limited effects on the problems of hospital patient care errors.

F. W. Ernst, M.D. — William G. Pace III, M. D.

Perhaps we as patients (yes, we physicians are patients, too) may need a patient advocate in the hospital with us around-the-clock. This person should question every medication given to us, every diagnostic test ordered, or any treatment rendered to us to help ensure no errors are being made. It is truly unfortunate that our healthcare system has come to this point.

IN SUMMARY

- Surgical and anesthesia patients should understand that hospital admission is not a "routine procedure" and that choosing the right hospital for surgery is a vital part of obtaining the highest quality of care.

- Hospital admission and length of stay are usually based on extent of care. There are four basic categories of admission: ambulatory, 23-hour care, direct admission, and emergency admission.

- Be sure to answer all questions during pre-admission interviews carefully and in adequate detail. Take the time to get it right!

CHAPTER TWO

SELECTING YOUR SURGEON

Dr. Pace

KEY POINT:

- **Never Assume That Your Surgeon Is an "Expert"—Take the Time and Trouble to Check Out His or Her Credentials and Experience.**

It's one of the most frightening—and one of the most promising—words in the English language: *surgery*. And it's a word that sooner or later confronts most of us as we grapple with the illnesses and other health problems that eventually catch up to just about everybody.

Most of the time, of course, surgery works in the service of health, and does a marvelous job of assisting us in the struggle to overcome our ailments. Whether the surgical procedure is aimed at relieving a chronic condition (gallstones, for example), or at repairing a sudden emergency disorder (appendicitis, perhaps, or a stroke-triggering blood clot), there's no doubt that it can be an effective weapon in the physician's arsenal—an efficient, high-tech tool that, properly used, can help you live a healthier life.

But surgery is also a frightening experience for most of us—there's simply no pretending about that—and such fears are perfectly understandable and appropriate. After all, who wouldn't feel a touch of anxiety when mulling the prospect of being "put to sleep" and then "cut on" in the service of better health?

Yes, undergoing surgery is a formidable assignment, no question about it. That's precisely why it's so important for you to choose the right surgeon—and a surgeon, above all, whom you can fully trust.

Make no mistake, here: when it comes to the extraordinarily serious business of allowing a medical professional to invade your body with a scalpel, you must establish that trust long before check-in day at the hospital!

For starters, you must determine—beyond even a scintilla of reasonable doubt—whether or not the surgeon to whom you've been referred actually possesses the training, the certification, and the vitally important on-the-job experience to manage your procedure with maximum skill and medical prudence.

Obviously, any failure to do your homework is simply unacceptable here; common sense, as well as good medical practice, requires that you become fully informed about the professional background of the surgeon you select.

Thankfully, most surgical procedures end quite successfully. But when they don't—and when needless tragedy is the result—it's often because the patient failed to accomplish the most important single task in surgery: determining the professional experience and competence of the surgeon.

Sadly enough, that's exactly what happened in the case of Brad Nathanson, a Florida retiree who paid a very high price for choosing the wrong surgeon. . .

****

For Brad Nathanson and his pal Mort, it was a daily ritual: first, they'd drop by Sal's Deli on Pompano Avenue for coffee and a bagel. Hunched over their cups of steaming java, the two retirees would gab furiously about their two favorite topics: the "mess in Washington" and their beloved Boston Red Sox.

"It's their karma," Brad would tell Mort, while spreading cream cheese on his onion bagel.

As always, the mustachioed Mort would glare at his buddy for a few seconds. Deadpan. Then, scowling: "Karma? What is this karma? The Red Sox don't have a left-handed stopper, you know that. They got from zero when it comes to pitching, period. That guy you read must be off his nut. . ."

The daily gab-fest! For Brad and Mort, two former office products salesmen who'd spent their careers calling on clients in and around Boston, retirement in Boca Raton meant a blessedly slow-paced existence . . . and a chance, finally, to settle back with that morning coffee and enjoy a few "war stories" with other men like themselves.

On the morning of September 10, 1997, however, as the two sat jawing away in their usual corner-booth, neither Brad nor Mort could have imagined that this would be the last time they'd ever share a table at Sal's.

"So," Mort growled at his fellow-retiree, as the two of them poured cream into their coffee, "you're finally gonna bite the bullet, huh, Brad?"

Nathanson, a tall, elegant-looking man whose snow-white hair was always perfectly combed, shook his head mournfully. "They're gonna do me tomorrow morning, Mort, over at Mercy. You know how it is with benign prostate—in and out, they take care of the enlargement, pow! I'll be home in a couple of days."

"Okay," said Mort carefully, "so no problem, huh?"

Brad stared at him. "No problem, Mort! I told you: they do this thing—this transurethral . . . whatever the hell it is. They do this stuff ten times a day! They just shrink the whole thing down: Bingo, no more pain in the prostate, and they tell me I'll be able to take a leak with the best of 'em! Hah!"

In spite of himself, Mort winced visibly, as he imagined the scalpel slicing into the incredibly sensitive area around the male prostate gland. But then he shook the vision off. "All right, my friend. Tell you what. I'll drop by Mercy, what, seven o'clock tomorrow night? Visiting hours? How about I bring you a vodka tonic?"

"I'll need it, Mort!"

The two of them laughed and finished their coffee. And then moments later, they were shaking hands and saying their farewells. It was the usual ritual, after which Brad would head for the small fishing pier that flanked his condominium. Maybe bait a hook or two and catch himself a red snapper for supper? Naaaah . . . not today. He was too nervous today.

In the end, he just sat for a couple of hours in a canvas chair that somebody had left on the pier. He watched a couple of younger guys trying to land a big sand shark one of then had hooked . . . but at the last moment the ugly, shovel-headed fish managed to break free and head for deeper water.

A lifelong bachelor, Brad Nathanson had remained very close to his sister, Ruth, who would be flying in from Atlanta later today, in order to help her 74-year-old brother through the admissions process and then remain at his bedside during the estimated two-day hospital stay.

Strictly routine. Because he didn't want to think about the whole business—didn't want to admit that he was afraid of the surgery, in fact—Brad Nathanson hadn't really taken the time to get to know his surgeon, Dr. Pitts. Hadn't Dr. Rosenfeld, the primary care physician at Brad's HMO, recommended him whole-heartedly? What the heck, they were all doctors . . . they were supposed to know what they were doing, right?

Besides, Dr. Pitts had seemed perfectly competent, totally professional during their one interview, three weeks before. Oh, maybe he was a little young, only about 35, but, hey, this was one of Florida's largest hospitals—they wouldn't let a guy conduct surgery, young or not, unless he knew what he was doing...

Routine.

The next morning, early, Brad's sister, Ruth Levin drove him to the big hospital on Winter Park Avenue to help him through the lengthy admitting process.

A short, energetic, high school biology teacher from Atlanta, Ruth kissed Brad on the cheek and patted his shoulder as they waited for the "routine" surgery to begin. Just before they began wheeling the patient toward the operating room, Dr. Pitts stepped through a doorway to greet them.

The youthful surgeon was smiling and rubbing his hands briskly together. "He'll do fine," he beamed at Ruth, "a resection like this—piece of cake!"

Frowning uneasily, Ruth nodded. Then she watched them wheel her brother down the gleaming hallway. . .

Unfortunately, however, what happened next was very far from being a "piece of cake."

As the medical evidence in a later malpractice case would clearly demonstrate, Dr. Pitts—along with his apparently incompetent anesthesiologist—failed to guard against one of the most obvious dangers in a "transurethral resection of the prostate" (a basic surgical technique aimed at reducing enlargement that is benign).

What the surgeon and the anesthesiologist somehow overlooked in this botched operation was the fact that when the patient's bladder is being inspected—via a small telescope inserted through the penis—the standard procedure is to irrigate a glycol-water solution into the bladder, to expand it and improve visibility, which means that, during an operation of any length, a great deal of this glycol-water solution can be absorbed into the blood.

The resulting danger can be described in a single word: hyponatremia, a condition in which the sodium in a patient's blood serum gradually drops to dangerously low levels because of dilution by the urologic irrigating solution.

To this day, no one at Mercy Hospital has managed to explain how the surgeon and the anesthesiologist (both were clearly responsible) failed to monitor Brad Nathanson's blood-sodium during what should have been routine surgery to shrink a benign prostate enlargement.

Perhaps the most egregious mistake of all, however, was what occurred after the operating-team witnessed the patient becoming extremely irritated and agitated under his spinal anesthetic. As every surgeon and anesthesiologist will tell you, such symptoms in the wake of a "spinal" can mean only two things:

1. The anesthetic, itself, has not been effective, or has begun to wear off;
2. The patient has become "hyponatremic", meaning that his blood-sodium-level has declined to the danger point.

The great danger in hyponatremia is that the victim will suffer irreversible brain damage.

Tragically, that is precisely the scenario that unfolded in the case of Brad Nathanson.

Two years later, the testimony in the giant malpractice case that Ruth Levin brought against both the hospital and the attending physicians made the consequences of this medical negligence appallingly clear.

For the unfortunate Mr. Nathanson, the days of critiquing the Boston Red Sox' pitching staff were gone forever. Having suffered the ghastliest health catastrophe imaginable—the only accurate phrase for it is "brain death"—the former salesman wound up in a full-time nursing care facility 40 miles from his former condo beside the Boca Raton fishing pier.

And his buddy, Mort? Although he managed to make the long trip to the nursing home now and then to visit his pal, Mort found the experience deeply saddening: each time he discovered his old friend sitting in a corner of the Dayroom, helpless and babbling.

****

Rx: How To Evaluate Your Surgeon

Would Brad Nathanson have enjoyed a better outcome if he had taken the time to get to know his surgical team's background and credentials better?

While no one can answer such hypothetical questions with absolute certainty, common sense tells us that such researching of the medical professionals we rely on can only help, in the effort to obtain the best surgical care available.

At first glance, of course, the task of choosing the right surgeon for your particular health problem seems daunting. What can a candidate for surgery expect, as he or she sets out to find the very best medical professional? Where do you go for information? To whom do you talk, and how much of what you hear should you believe?

It all sounds rather overwhelming at first. But if you slow for a minute, and take a deep breath, you'll quickly see that you can break the job down into a few fairly simple, easy steps.

For starters, let's talk for a few minutes about the two key yardsticks you will be using in evaluating any surgeon's bona fides: his training and his credentials. And let's be quite up-front about this:

regardless of the Declaration of Independence, all surgeons are not created equal!

Wouldn't it be nice if they were, and all you had to do to find the ideal surgeon was "flip through the Yellow Pages?"

It's astonishing to think about how little the general public really knows about the training and background of surgeons, or about the requirements and the standards in force at the various hospitals where these technicians employ their skills.

Still, any potential surgery patient can learn a great deal simply by examining the surgeon's credentials. Obviously, finding out where he or she earned a medical degree and then did a surgical residency can tell you a lot about qualifications. Of course, acceptance ratios at medical schools vary from institution to institution. For example, at Harvard, a prestigious medical facility, only one applicant in about 200 will be accepted. (Note: Many potential applicants don't apply for admission believing that their chances of being accepted are simply too low.)

According to recent surveys, only about ten percent of those who apply to American medical schools are accepted.

Question 1: What happens to the rest of this great swarm of applicants?

Answer: If they've got the money to foot the bill, many will wind up in a foreign country—in Mexico, Grenada, or Italy, or one of the new schools just opening its doors in Eastern Europe.

Question 2: Is the education that takes place on these distant campuses the equivalent of the education in an accredited American medical school? I don't know the answer to that question. And yet it's also true that I have never met a physician who chose one of these foreign schools over an accredited American school to which he or she had also been admitted!

While medical schools may vary in quality, so do surgical residency programs. Many of these residencies are controlled by the

National Matching Plan, which tries to link new medical school grads to the right hospital by assessing hospital size, the size and quality of the teaching staff, and the quality of the teaching that actually goes on at any particular institution.

Yet the bottom line remains the same: there are always many more applications than positions in surgical residencies. And those who don't receive a surgical residency slot do have other options available: they can go into one of the many other branches of medicine, or they can seek a residency in an unapproved program in this country or overseas.

But there's a catch, and an important one: those who do settle for the "unapproved" residency program will not be eligible to apply for board certification.

To understand why that matters, we need to ask: what is board certification, anyway?

The process actually began in 1916, when a number of surgeons from the U.S. (and later Canada) formed a "fellowship" to promote improved quality of surgical standards and continuing education.

In those earlier days, surgical education was based much more on a kind of "on-the-job" apprenticeship model than it is today, and it was often considered fashionable to go to Vienna or other European centers for special training, especially for those who were specializing in "ENT" (ear, nose, and throat) surgery. Through the 1920s however, there was no formal accreditation or certification process.

By 1930, surgical practice was becoming more mature and sophisticated—but the various training programs were far from uniform in teaching methods and content. All too often, the trainee was simply used as cheap labor, and paid nothing.

(Example: My own salary during my first year of surgical training in Philadelphia in 1953 consisted of a free room—shared with a roommate—and meals in the cafeteria. Later, my group of four interns won a hefty raise—from $0 to $50 a month for each of us!)

Responding to the need for standards, then, professors of surgery from around the country gathered in the 1930s to outline what they regarded as the "nucleus of knowledge" for the practicing surgeon. They also created an examination that would lead to "certification" in surgery.

At the outset, this "board certification" was offered on a "grandfather basis" to those who were judged to be practicing high-quality surgery, already—while the standard certification was awarded only after an examination. As you might expect, the introduction of these new standards triggered some amusing complications. In one celebrated instance, a New York surgeon refused to accept board certification as an initial member.

Many years later, when he discovered that such certification had become extremely important, he contacted the board to announce that he would now "accept" their offer. And when he was told that the examination would now be required, the crusty old medico snapped, "Who could possibly examine me?"

These days, board certification is required for staff privileges at most hospitals. Be careful, however: it is never safe to assume that a physician is board-certified. And to complicate the problem even further, it's also true there are over 100 "boards" that aren't even recognized by the American Board of Medical Specialists (ABMS).

It's important to understand, here, that there are only 24 recognized specialty boards, and that some of the others require only an "application fee" for membership—after which they will supply a very impressive-looking document for the office wall!

Although the ABMS offices are located in Philadelphia, you don't have to go there to check on your surgeon's credentials. Most public libraries have a copy of the *Directory of American Medical Specialists*. Published by Marquis (also the publishers of *Who's Who*), the Directory lists not only those 24 approved boards, but also the thousands of surgical specialists now at work in the U.S. Each one is identified by name, birthday, medical school, residency, hospital affiliations, and, usually, telephone numbers. (Unavoidably, there are occasional errors in such massive listings, but I've found only one omission in 25 years of using this tool, and it was promptly corrected.)

Next question: what happens to those surgeons who fail the board exams, or don't take them at all? As medical doctors, of course, they still have several options. They can always continue to practice under the preceptorship of another surgeon, if the hospital will permit it. It's also true that at some non-accredited hospitals, surgeons lacking board certification may practice, but such a step will put the hospital at greater risk if the surgeon commits malpractice.

Another option for the non-certified physician is to accept a position in an emergency room (even though he or she may not have certification in Emergency Medicine, either). The surgeon may also choose to practice as part of a group, earning a handsome salary, but the long-term future for that kind of occupation is limited for most physicians. Usually, the best single option is to continue to study for the board exams, and to re-take them in the future.

Still, there are some other possible options for our non-certified surgeon. Although not trained as a general practitioner, the candidate may choose to enter "general practice." Of course, he or she will not then be eligible to take the Family Practice Board Examinations—and as that specialty gains in prestige, a failure to hold those boards may preclude the physician from practicing that specialty as well.

Another approach is for the surgeon to simply join one of the over 100 non-certified "boards," which supply him with the impressive papering for the wall, and not much else. So the surgical patient must beware: when selecting a physician, ask to see his credentials—or go to the library and document them fully, yourself!

It's no accident, of course, that when physicians end up in a courtroom trial of malpractice, the subject of "board certification" usually becomes a crucial part of the debate.

That's when you'll hear the defense attorney asking, "Is board certification always necessary for the performance of safe surgery?" The lawyer is hoping to hear the word "no," as you might expect, but the correct answer isn't a simple yes or no. As any good "expert witness" in this area will testify, practicing surgery without board certification isn't the same as driving your car without a license! (After all, you can operate a vehicle safely, if you choose, even if you're without a license.)

Remember, then, when thinking about the business of certification: there are only three reasons why a doctor isn't certified:

1. He or she isn't eligible to take the boards (perhaps because of lack of residency program accreditation, or because the director of same refused to certify the participant as a safe surgeon).
2. The candidate failed the boards one or more times.
3. The candidate was simply too lazy (or making too much money at the time) to bother with taking the exams.

But let us be crystal-clear on this point: both Dr. Ernst and I strongly recommend that you do not seek treatment of any kind (and especially of the surgical kind) from a non-certified physician.

While there's no guarantee that a board-certified physician won't make a mistake or commit malpractice, the odds are infinitely better for a good outcome, because your physician will have better knowledge and better training than a non-certified counterpart.

In recent years, an increasing number of state medical boards have adopted a physician-profiling system which is available to the public. These physician profiles will only contain information referable to the physicians' practice in any particular state. For example, if a physician is presently practicing in Florida, his/her Florida profile will not contain any information from any other state in which that physician may have practiced.

This is one valuable source of information when you are trying to check up on a particular physician's credentials. At the present time, 25 states have a relatively complete profiling system while the other 25 states either have no system in place or the system in place has only limited information available to the public.

The Federation of State Medical Boards located in Euless, TX, has opened its Physician Data Center for public inquiries. The Federation offers access to physician-specific information including board disciplinary actions taken by any state medical board in the U.S. or its territories. There is a $9.95 charge per query. Its website for this information is: www.docinfo.org

IN SUMMARY

- Never assume that your surgeon is an "expert." Take the time and trouble to check out his/her credentials and experience.

- Do some research, and make sure that the surgeon who will be performing your operation is "board certified."

F. W. Ernst, M.D. — William G. Pace III, M. D.

Approved Specialty Boards

The following is a listing of the twenty-four boards comprising the membership of the America Board of Medical Specialists.

1. The American Board of Allergy and Immunology, (A conjoint Board of the American Board of Internal Medicine and the American Board of Pediatrics) Inc., Philadelphia, PA.
2. The America Board of Anesthesiology, Inc., Raleigh, NC.
3. The American Board of Colon and Rectal Surgery, Inc., Taylor, MI.
4. The American Board of Dermatology, Inc., Detroit, MI.
5. The American Board of Emergency Medicine, Inc., East Lansing, MI.
6. The American Board of Family Practice, Inc., Lexington, KY
7. The American Board of Internal Medicine, Inc., Philadelphia, PA.
8. The American Board of Neurological Surgery, Inc., Houston, TX.
9. The American Board of Medical Genetics Inc., Bethesda, MD.
10. The America Board of Nuclear Medicine, Inc., St. Louis, MO
11. The American Board of Obstetrics and Gynecology, Inc., Dallas, TX
12. The American Board of Ophthalmology, Inc., Bala Cynwyd, PA.
13. The American Board of Orthopedic Surgery, Inc., Chapel Hill, NC.
14. The American Board of Otolaryngology, Inc., Houston, TX
15. The American Board of Pathology, Inc., Tampa, FL
16. The American Board of Pediatrics, Inc., Chapel Hill, NC
17. The American Board of Physical Medicine and Rehabilitation, Inc., Rochester, MN

18. The American Board of Plastic Surgery, Inc., Philadelphia, PA
19. The American Board of Preventative Medicine, Inc., Chicago, IL
20. The American Board of Psychiatry and Neurology, Inc., Deerfield, IL
21. The American Board of Radiology, Inc., Tucson, AZ
22. The American Board of Surgery, Inc., Chicago, IL
23. The American Board of Thoracic Surgery, Inc., Evanston, IL
24. The America Board of Urology, Inc., Charlottesville, VA

To check on Board Certification Status: 1-866-275-2267

F. W. Ernst, M.D. — William G. Pace III, M. D.

Truth, Lies and the OR

CHAPTER THREE

ANESTHESIA-CARE PROVIDERS:
"Who Will Watch Over Me While I Sleep?"

Dr. Ernst

KEY POINT:

- **In order to receive the very best possible medical care, surgical patients should ask as many questions about their anesthesia (and about the credentials and qualifications of their anesthesia deliverers) as they ask about the surgical procedure itself!**

The alarm clock went off promptly at six a.m.: *Clanngghhh!*

Butch Shockett opened one eye . . . then fumbled for the switch that would turn the damn thing off. But a moment later his brother Todd was looming above his canvas cot.

"Come on, Tiger!" roared Todd. "We got some squirrels to run down!"

Ten minutes later, the two Shockett brothers—both in their late 20s and from Greenbriar, a small Tennessee town about 80 miles from Chattanooga—were sitting at the wooden table in their mountain cabin.

It was a bright, blue Saturday morning in early June of 1999. The "Shockett boys" were in the middle of one of their beloved hunting trips. And now, as they sat pouring skim milk over their bowls of oatmeal, they were engaged in their favorite pastime: mocking each other's hunting skills.

"If I was you," laughed Todd, as he reached for the plastic squeeze-bottle of honey, "I wouldn't even bother to bring that shotgun along today."

"Since you don't know how to use it, why don't you just throw rocks at them squirrels?"

Butch Shockett, a stocky, freckled young man with baby-blue eyes and a booming laugh, gave his brother a hard shove. "Shut that yap, brother, before I put this size-10 hunting boot up next to your tonsils!" The two of them roared, and Butch picked up the squeeze-bottle.

But then he caught himself: "Whoops! The doc told me no more sugar—not even any honey on the oatmeal!"

Butch had been diagnosed with moderate Type II diabetes about eight months before. Although Dr. Blasingame at Mercy Medical hadn't required him to take daily insulin injections, the doctor was concerned: Butch's glucose tests showed that he was right on the edge of serious diabetes.

Under the doctor's stern new regimen, the fun-loving Butch had already lost more than 20 pounds. He was watching his diet carefully, these days—no more of those chocolate snack cakes he loved to wolf down with lunch! And he was also working out hard, every other day, as part of Dr. Blasingame's recommended new exercise program.

So far, the disease seemed to be under control . . . although Butch sometimes felt a bit shaky, a bit dizzy after meals, and he sometimes woke up in the middle of the night with a raging thirst, and then gulped what seemed like gallons of cold water straight from the tap.

Still, everybody knew that Type II, or "Adult Onset," diabetes progresses very slowly over the patient's lifetime: as long as Butch remained careful about his diet and got his exercise, he could go to work every day (he drove a big tractor out at the Stanton Strip-Mine) without having to take those miserable damn insulin shots.

Now he slapped the honey bottle back on the table. "Let's go get them squirrels, you dipstick!"

Within 25 minutes, they were making their way along Polecat Hollow, a narrow stream valley overhung with windblown mountain sassafras and shaggy red gum branches.

Carrying identical Remington double-barreled shotguns, the two hadn't seen a single squirrel yet—was the entire world still asleep?

"There!"

Todd was pointing to the higher branches of a tall sycamore, where a fat, furry tail could be seen twitching, twitching...

Butch nodded. Flipping the safety-catch off his trigger, he began to move in closer. Soon he was easing himself over a tall oak log that blocked the trail.

Then it happened.

Butch's right boot hit a slick patch of wet lichen on the side of the log—in a flash, he'd lost his footing.

Down he went. The shotgun flew from his hands. And as Butch fell, the butt of the Remington banged hard against a nearby tree stump POW!

The shotgun had discharged and Butch was hit!

In a moment, Todd was leaning above him. "Oh, my God..." The bright red blood was already streaming down Butch's leg. Todd could see where the blast had taken out a big piece of his brother's hip, before ripping into his abdomen!

The next hour was an agony for both brothers. Sweating and grunting with effort, Todd fought his way out of Polecat Hollow with his bleeding brother on his back. Abandoning the shotguns and other supplies on the trail, Todd raced to get Butch to the emergency room at Barclay Hospital, the nearest medical facility, located about 15 miles down county Road "B" at McKesson.

By now covered with blood himself, the furiously panting Todd Shockett lurched into the ER while screaming, "He's been shot! He's been shot!"

The four-member medical staff at work in this tiny rural hospital instantly jumped into action. While the local surgeon hurried toward the facility from a nearby golf course, his Certified Registered Nurse Anesthetist (CRNA) began asking Butch a series of standard questions.

Did the accident victim suffer from any serious allergies? Had he ever been diagnosed with heart disease? Epilepsy? Had he ever undergone an appendectomy?

Suddenly, however, right in the middle of a question, the freckled young hunter began to bellow with pain, "Damn . . . my hip!"

Now the CRNA turned to Todd, who was standing nearby.

"You're his brother? Help me finish these! Has he ever had a reaction to an antibiotic? Any history of drug or alcohol abuse? Any fainting spells or convulsions after meals?"

But then, just as she was in the middle of asking him "Any history of diabetes?", the arriving surgeon came hurrying through the door. Because Todd was eager to talk to him, and was only half-listening to the CRNA, and because his answer to all of the previous questions had been "no", he absent-mindedly shook his head in response to the query about diabetes.

A moment later, the CRNA had finished the questionnaire and flung it aside, and was helping the surgeon to begin preparing the patient for exploratory surgery.

What followed was a very unfortunate example of what can happen when an anesthesia provider fails to prepare adequately for surgery.

In fact, Butch Shockett had suffered only a deep flesh wound: through a nearly miraculous fluke of physics, the shotgun pellets had ripped the tissue around his liver to shreds (while also breaking his hip-bone in three places), but hadn't actually damaged the vital organ—a fact which the exploratory surgery soon revealed.

And, although the shooting victim had lost slightly more than a pint of blood, the wound had safely sealed itself by now; Butch was in no real danger of bleeding to death.

Ironically, the only significant physical danger that Butch Shockett now faced was the exploratory surgery itself!

As it turned out, his diabetes had been rapidly worsening in the weeks that led up to the accident—a fact which the over-stressed, under-attentive CRNA had failed to catch, because she made a classic mistake in preparing patients for anesthesia: she had failed to get the patient (or a family member or close friend) to sit down calmly and talk about each of her "pre-op" questions in careful detail, in order to build a careful, accurate medical profile.

In the case of Butch Shockett, that mistake nearly proved fatal.

Because his blood chemistry had been considerably altered by the administration of general anesthesia, Butch's blood sugar had rapidly soared toward the danger-point, a condition that was of course masked by the anesthesia.

But not for long.

As Butch was sitting up in bed in the recovery room, and listening to the good news from the surgeon, he suddenly began to drift into what would be a nearly lethal diabetic convulsion.

For the next six hours, the doctors and nurses at the Barclay Hospital would fight to get the young hunter's snarled blood chemistry back under control—while the CRNA who had failed to uncover the diabetes in the pre-op interview berated herself for what had been a potentially fatal mistake.

Luckily, Butch Shockett survived this close brush with anesthesia-triggered brain convulsions, and was soon back in the hills of Tennessee, chasing rabbits and squirrels through Polecat Hollow once again. But the chilling memory of what had happened at Barclay Hospital would be with him for a lifetime.

****

Rx: How To Evaluate Anesthesia-Care Providers

With stark clarity, the medical file on Butch Shockett illustrates a key fact about modern medicine: patients who undergo surgery must be just as careful about choosing their anesthesia-care provider as they are about choosing the surgeon who will perform their operation.

To understand why that's true, let's step back for a moment to make a few general observations about anesthesia and surgery.

First of all, it's now clear that over the past three decades or so, the general public has become increasingly aware of the medical specialty of anesthesia, and of its crucial importance in protecting patient safety.

Along with this increased awareness, there is a growing body of knowledge today about the dangers of anesthetic complications and also—to the discredit of the medical profession—about some recent, notorious abuses of patient-care by anesthesia personnel.

In order to understand just what goes on during anesthesia, it's helpful to identify the various medical professionals involved in the process.

Let's start with the anesthesiologist (MDA), who is a physician, a graduate from a medical school with a degree in medicine or osteopathic medicine. He or she then completes a minimum of four years of postgraduate training in an anesthesia residency educational program. At least three of these four years will be focused on the specialty of anesthesia. During the fourth year, the anesthesiologist will concentrate on a sub-specialty that might include (but not be limited to) pediatric, obstetric, cardiac, intensive care, or pain management.

After the successful completion of a residency program approved by the American Board of Medical Specialists, an anesthesiologist is considered "board-eligible." This term indicates that he or she has earned the right to sit for the written-exam section of the American Board of Anesthesiologists' (ABA's) certification process.

Once a candidate has passed the written exam, he or she is eligible to sit for the oral portion of the test, which usually occurs about one year later. After that, if successful, the anesthesiologist will be board-certified and named a "diplomate" of the ABA.

As of January 1, 2000, all certifications awarded by the ABA are time-limited to ten years and, thus, will expire ten years after being issued. Such a change means that, in order to be recertified by the ABA, an anesthesiologist will have to repeat the certification process every ten years. The ABA has chosen this step in order to reassure the public that anesthesiologists will be required to maintain their qualifications in the future.

At present, certification by the ABA is the only such physician-certification available in the United States. (Several sub-specialty certifications are available under ABA procedures.)

So much for the anesthesiologist. The next player on the anesthesia-care team is the Certified Registered Nurse Anesthetist (CRNA), a registered nurse who has earned a Bachelor of Science degree in nursing, then spent an additional year in critical care nursing, followed by an average of 28 months of training in anesthesia (ranging from 24-33 months). After the training is complete, each candidate must pass a national exam in order to become certified.

Next in the lineup is the Anesthesia Assistant (AA). This medical professional must have a Bachelor of Science degree as a prerequisite to beginning anesthesia training. Such training, as in the case of the CRNA, ranges from 24-28 months in length, and once again, upon completion, the candidate must pass a written national qualifying examination in order to practice anesthesia as a licensed AA. This exam differs from the one taken by the CRNA. And there's one other difference, as well: the AA can enter anesthesia training without any nursing or medical school background.

It's important to point out here that the CRNA always possesses a nursing education background, while the anesthesiologist invariably has an extensive background in medical training. Both professionals receive similar basic anesthesia training—except in the areas of pharmacology, pathophysiology, physiology, and internal medicine.

In spite of this difference in background, the CRNA is quite capable of practicing anesthesia with medical supervision by someone other than an MDA, and the law allows this as well. In these cases, as a matter of fact, the physician ultimately responsible for the supervision of the CRNA is the surgeon, although in some situations an obstetrician, a dentist, a podiatrist or some other MD may fill this role.

It's also true that the majority of surgical residencies include little if any anesthesia training, although a few programs offer a six-month rotation in anesthesia. Consequently, most surgeons have limited knowledge about anesthesia—and especially about the various complications and treatments that are involved in administering it. If an anesthetic complication arises that is beyond the expertise of the CRNA involved, the chances are that it will also be beyond the expertise of the surgeon, a situation which can trigger a medical predicament.

Generally speaking, you'll find these solo CRNAs at work in smaller hospitals or in semi-rural areas. Given the harsh economics of medicine today, it's simply not feasible for these smaller facilities to hire both an MDA and a CRNA. Let's face it: as a critical area of care, anesthesia does benefit from the advantages offered by a larger, more fully staffed hospital environment.

As for the AA, who owns the sketchiest medical background: these professionals are only allowed to practice their craft under the supervision of an MDA. And the AAs are not even licensed in all states. Currently you'll find that there are only five training facilities for AAs in the U.S.—compared to more than 108 programs for nurse anesthetists.

Of course, a good anesthesia-delivery care team can consist of various combinations of these specialists, depending on circumstances. Today, you'll find that the "anesthesia-care team" concept is most prevalent. Such a configuration calls for an MDA supervising CRNAs or AAs or a combination of both. The main advantage in this approach is that two caregivers trained in anesthesia are involved with each patient, as opposed to only one—which is what happens when an MDA or CRNA works independently.

Remember, though, that—as happens in all professions—there are some MDAs and some CRNAs who are extremely well qualified, dedicated, and equally capable of functioning on an independent basis. And there are some of each who are less qualified, skillful, and committed to the profession, and thus fail to meet the highest standards of quality care.

My own preference, when it comes to choosing the right care provider, is the team approach in which the CRNAs work closely with the MDAs. (Indeed, that's the system that I've relied on throughout my own career as an anesthesiologist.)

Next step: it's important to understand, when you're making decisions about your anesthesia-care team, that it's acceptable—for insurance billing purposes—for an MDA to supervise up to four anesthesia procedures simultaneously in the same geographic location. However, it's also true that there are no restrictions or specific guidelines as to what types of procedures take place in those rooms. Nor do the regulations take into account the seriousness of the surgery, its potential complications, or the medical condition of the patient. The supervision ratio when residents and/or student nurse anesthetists are involved is 1:2.

The question of how many rooms an MDA will supervise is best left to the personal discretion and judgment of the MDA.

Obviously, the amount of time that gets spent on each patient will depend on the number of anesthesia cases the MDA is supervising—along with the relative difficulty of the procedures and the commitment of the MDA to quality care. Realistically, there's always the danger that the MDA will spread himself too thinly, posing a real threat to optimum care for each patient. And, of course, it's also true that the more anesthesia procedures an MDA supervises, the lower the overhead costs and the greater the profits! (But make no mistake: it's strictly illegal and unethical for an MDA to supervise simultaneous anesthesia procedures at geographically separate institutions.)

Although there are a number of hospitals around the country that offer training programs in anesthesia, only a small percentage of them will train both anesthesia residents and nurse anesthetists or anesthesia assistants. And that means that if you're a patient in a teaching hospital, you might very well wind up with a trainee on your anesthesia team.

Remember that the training level and type of supervision can affect the level of care. Remember also that there are no specific guidelines for the "one-to-four ratio" in supervision when nurse anesthetists, or anesthesia assistants are involved in the anesthesia care.

Another key aspect of American surgery today is the concept of "outpatient" (or one-day) surgery, which began to be popularized in this country—starting in 1969—by Wallace A. Reed, MD. By the mid-1990's, the practice had grown to the point that more than half of all surgery was ambulatory. Today, 75% of all surgery is one-day surgery.and 25% of all surgery is office-based surgery. When surgery occurs in the doctor's office and the anesthesia employed consists of intravenous sedation, there may not be a qualified, trained specialist in anesthesia present to monitor the level of the sedation and the vital signs. On the other hand, obviously, the use of general anesthesia would require trained, qualified anesthesia personnel, under the present-day standard of care.

So much for the basics about the anesthesia care providers. The next question is: how can you best use this information when you find yourself confronting surgery and anesthesia?

First, you should prepare yourself for—and insist on—a pre-operative visit by a member of the anesthesia department. Here you will be asked questions about your medical history and your past anesthesia history, before a careful description of the type of anesthesia planned for you is presented.

You'll also be given a chance to ask questions. Here is your opportunity to discuss your questions about anesthesia, along with fears and concerns. This is also the perfect time to identify the composition of your anesthesia-care team and make any requests of them.

Remember: if you prefer not to have a trainee work on your case, say so! Also, if you're concerned about the MDA "supervision ratio," be sure to find out how many other procedures the MDA will be supervising while your own surgery is underway. If you don't like what you hear, then make your own recommendation about the ratio. You're paying for this, and you have a perfect right to demand the best care available.

Also ask if the medical professional who conducts the pre-operative anesthesia evaluation will be the same one who performs the anesthesia. Or will the evaluator also serve as the anesthesia supervisor? It's important to understand that, on some occasions, the evaluator may not actually be working on your case. There are many reasons to account for this, including:

- The operating room may be quite busy, with frequent changes in scheduling, making it impossible to fully control the personnel involved.

- Unavoidable delays (longer-than-expected surgical procedures, for example) may affect scheduling.
- The anesthesia personnel who makes the pre-op visits may not be scheduled to work the next day.

Regardless, the anesthesia evaluator should communicate your requests or other concerns to the anesthesia personnel who will actually be working on your case.

If this pre-operative visit is omitted, or you don't get satisfactory answers to your questions, you should refuse to take pre-op medicine or to proceed with surgery until these issues are resolved.

During the first 48 hours after your surgery, you should expect a post-op visit from a member of the anesthesia department. If your surgery was "one-day," this visit will probably consist of a phone call from a staffer at the outpatient facility. The visit gives you a chance to discuss any questions or complications arising from the anesthesia procedure. It's also a chance to air any final questions, or express any criticisms or complaints. And yes, we do appreciate a "thank you" now and then!

Remember: if you do experience any anesthesia complications—such as an allergic reaction or other abnormal response to a drug, or lung problems, or even cardiac difficulty—it's very important for you to completely understand what went wrong. One helpful strategy is to keep a written summary of the pertinent points for future reference. (Many times you can prevent another such anesthesia problem by taking care of it in advance, provided you know about it.)

One other key area in the world of anesthesia is emergency surgery. Now, emergencies may occur at any time, but the term generally refers to procedures accomplished between 11 p.m. and 6 a.m. What usually happens during these periods is that the anesthesia will be administered by personnel on night-call; obviously, your choices in personnel will be minimal. But don't forget that if you have a reasonable objection to being treated by an anesthesia provider you can't communicate with, you can probably postpone that surgery, at least temporarily, and request another provider.

Currently in the U.S., it is standard procedure to have a CRNA or an MDA (or both) on call in the hospital overnight. Still, this may not be the case in small outlying and rural hospitals. You might wish to inquire about this if you're suddenly facing the prospect of emergency surgery. Remember, too, that at some hospitals the MDA still takes calls from home—and may even direct the CRNA to do the emergency procedure alone, while the MDA remains at home

But emergency surgery is definitely one area where the patient benefits greatly from having two pairs of experienced hands at work on his anesthesia!

Remember that it's not uncommon for anesthesia personnel who have taken a call the night before to be working on anesthesia procedures the next day. (They will frequently remain on hand until the work load lightens and the MDA releases them for that day.) Obviously, if these personnel have had little or no sleep, their performance could be affected. Find out! Just how much rest has your anesthesia provider obtained the night before? If you don't like the answer, you and your family may need to make a judgment call as to whether or not you're willing to proceed. And if you aren't, you've got a perfect right to request a personnel change.

After reading this chapter, you ought to fully understand how anesthesia care is delivered in this country . . . and you should be able to answer the crucial question: "Who will watch over me while I sleep?"

Good luck with your surgery . . . and your anesthesia!

F. W. Ernst, M.D. — William G. Pace III, M. D.

IN SUMMARY

- In order to receive the very best possible medical care, surgical patients should ask as many questions about their anesthesia—and about the credentials and qualifications of their anesthesia-deliverers—as they ask about the surgical procedure itself.

- You can improve your chances for high-quality anesthesia care enormously by knowing all the members of your anesthesia-care team and their functions during surgery, as outlined in this chapter.

- Take full advantage of your pre-operative visit with the anesthesia team to ask all of the questions you can, while outlining your own special needs and problems.

CHAPTER FOUR

PREPARING CHILDREN FOR SURGERY:
"I Am Not a Small Adult!"

Dr. Ernst

KEY POINT:

- **Medical professionals and parents alike need to understand one vitally important thing about preparing children for surgery: the kids are not merely small adults who are about to undergo an operation. In fact, they require an entirely different regimen of patient care, from admitting to departure.**

The nightmare would haunt me for more than 20 years.

Picture the scene: a lonely stretch of railroad tracks in the middle of a vast, featureless desert. As far as the eye can see, nothing but blowing sand and withered scrub brush. . .

And here he comes.

A tiny child, four years old, is running frantically along the tracks . . . running as hard as he can, but losing ground with every step. The train is pulling away from him.

"Momma! Momma!"

But it's no use. No matter how fast he runs, he can't catch that train. And now, his eyes burning with horror and fear, he watches his mother waving to him from the last car of the receding train, watches her tiny figure grow smaller and smaller, shrinking down to a doll-like image that gradually vanishes—

POW!--his right foot slams against a railroad tie, and down he goes, tumbling head over heels, falling helplessly into the deep, black pit of yawning space that waits to devour him. . .

A moment later, however, I suddenly wake up.

I sit bolt-upright in the bed, heart hammering, cold sweat popping out all along my forehead. Easy, easy, it was only a dream! I sit there, staring at the bedside clock. It's 4:30 in the morning, a summer morning in 1964, and I'm a 24-year-old medical student—and yet I'm still struggling with the effects of this childhood trauma!

****

Shakespeare got it right, as always, when he had Prospero declare, in "The Tempest," that nightmares are quite revealing of the psychological trauma that sooner or later afflicts every human being: "We are such stuff as dreams are made of, and our little life is rounded with a sleep!"

Let me tell you quite candidly that it took several years of counseling—and a great deal of inner soul-searching—before Dr. Fred Ernst finally came to terms with the demons that had haunted him since age four, when the surgical removal of his tonsils and adenoids triggered a devastating psychological trauma.

The year of that operation was 1944, and I was scared half to death.

How well I remember that grim, rainy morning when we set out for the hospital, at 6 a.m., in order to be ready for "outpatient" surgery at 8 a.m.!

And how well I remember the terror that I felt, at the moment when the orderly took me from my parents and led me toward the elevators. Suddenly, I was entirely on my own. A child of four, I would have to cope somehow with the strange clothes they were putting on me, and with the terrifying medical equipment that beeped and glittered so threateningly from every corner.

Can you imagine the fear and abandonment that this little child endured?

I remember sitting on the stretcher outside the operating room, curled into a shivering ball of fear, and listening to the unfamiliar sounds of a busy hospital . . . including the sound of several other children weeping hysterically for their mothers, somewhere nearby.

Amazingly enough, however, not a single person stopped by to ask how I was doing, or to provide a moment of gentle comfort.

After what seemed an eternity, a nurse finally arrived to escort me into the operating room. Off we went—without a word of explanation from anybody about what was going to happen next, or what I might expect.

A moment later, I was struggling through the worst agony I'd ever known in my short life: the ghastly moment when they lowered that dark, stinking mask over my face. Restrained on the table, and unable to resist, I gagged and fought for air.

A moment later, my horrified screams were cut short by the arrival of the worst odor I'd ever experienced—the hellish aroma of scorched, rotting fur—as the "drop ether" that they used for general anesthesia in those days slowly took effect.

Struggling frantically, I heard my own screams die off one by one, as I fell into the black hole of the Train Nightmare, and watched my mother vanish down the tracks…

The aftermath of this grisly experience would be long-lasting and quite harmful to me. Soon after returning home from the surgery, I would begin to experience stark terror at the sound of a shrieking fire engine or ambulance.

As you might expect, my parents did their best to help me work through these fears, by reading children's books about fire trucks and even taking me on a tour of the local firehouse in order to show me how kind and friendly the firemen were. My mom also made arrangements for me to drop by the local doctor's office, in the hope that a pleasing, peaceful "visit to the doctor" might ease my terrible fears.

But these measures turned out to be too little, too late.

By the time I reached kindergarten, this irrational fear of doctors and hospitals had reached alarming proportions. Quickly I came to fear the school's required trips to the school clinic for routine physical exams, eye-tests, and inoculations. Indeed, so great was my terror of anything having to do with medicine, that I would quickly run to the bathroom and lock myself in at the first announcement of an impending clinic-visit.

As any good psychologist could have pointed out, all of these fears were directly linked to the nightmare of my tonsillectomy.

Incredible as it may sound, I was in medical school myself before I finally managed to conquer those brutal fears.

I am also convinced that it was my growing professional knowledge about both surgery and anesthesia that allowed me to overcome the night terrors that had afflicted me ever since I was a four-year-old!

It's been more than 60 years now since that small child cried out on the operating table. But I think the story is still worth telling, because the danger that psychological trauma will be inflicted on children during surgical procedures is just as real today as it ever was. And make no mistake: when such painful injury overtakes an innocent child, it's usually because the medical personnel involved lack knowledge and understanding of—or concern for—the tender psyches of children.

Truth, Lies and the OR

****

Rx: How to Prepare Little Ones for Surgery

To understand how such damage to these little ones can occur, it's useful to examine the work of David Vernon, a psychologist whose pediatric studies in the 1960s broke new ground in our knowledge about childhood "separation anxiety."

In a particularly compelling article, "The Changes in Children's Behavior After Hospitalization," Mr. Vernon pointed out that pediatric patients between the ages of 6 and 48 months are the ones most adversely affected by hospitalization and illness.

In addition, he outlined how the relationship between behavior and hospitalization powerfully affects the psychological trauma that always attends parent-child separation to one degree or another. Labeling the fear "separation anxiety," Mr. Vernon described how the child's fear of losing parental protection can be triggered in the hospital setting, especially among the slightly older children who are clearly able to recognize that their mothers or fathers have "vanished" during key periods in a hospitalization.

Mr. Vernon's research was especially valuable in describing the inner reactions of children who, in order to undergo surgery, are first taken from their parents and then dispatched to an operating room where anesthesia will be administered—an area that the researcher defined as the "hostile hospital environment."

Mr. Vernon's outstanding contribution, like that of many other dedicated pediatric researchers, helps us understand how medical professionals and parents can best assist children in dealing with this separation anxiety. For starters, say the researchers, it's important to find ways to keep the separation time to an absolute minimum whenever the child is awake.

F. W. Ernst, M.D. — William G. Pace III, M. D.

This rule of thumb means that parents should be allowed to stay with their children until the anesthesia personnel are ready to escort the child into the operating room—where they should be prepared to begin the anesthesia induction immediately. Usually, that step is easiest to achieve in an outpatient facility, where the pre-operative waiting areas and the operating suites are located in the same area. Of course, the process is more difficult in a hospital environment, where the patient's room and the operating room will probably be found on different floors.

However, the one thing parents and medical professionals can control here is the time frame—and it's crucially important to make sure that there is minimal delay between the time the child leaves the parents and the anesthesia induction begins.

To help the child most, we also need to look at the time frame required in the post-anesthesia recovery room. The sooner a child can be reunited with parents post-operatively, the less chance for the development of separation anxiety. It's interesting to note that, these days, there is a growing trend among anesthesia departments to allow parents into the recovery room to help with post-operative care.

Because the logistics are simpler, such flexible visiting arrangements for parents seem easier to organize at the outpatient surgery facility than in the typical hospital.

Parents should also be aware that they have a right to request special procedures and schedules that will lessen the danger of separation anxiety in their children.

So, attention, all parents: don't be discouraged by that authoritative-sounding "Our policy does not include that accommodation!" Stand tall, and don't allow such blanket statements to prevent you from doing all you can to protect your child's psychic health, by making any reasonable request—or seeking any reasonable compromise—that you think is warranted by the circumstances.

Truth, Lies and the OR

Another useful tool in the campaign to keep your little ones from psychological trauma during surgery is pre-operative education. Parents can choose from a huge variety of children's books about hospitals and surgery, all of which do their best to make the experience as unthreatening and positive as possible. I strongly urge parents to read at least one of these books with their child, well in advance of the scheduled surgery.

It's also extremely important that the parents not lie to their children about any aspect of the surgical experience. Such deception not only erodes the parents' credibility, but it can also provoke distrust in the child of medical personnel, and adults in general.

As for the child's experience with anesthesia, I hope that my earlier description of the terrors I endured under that ether mask will convince one and all that there's simply no reason for kids to be forced into this nightmare.

Certainly, one of the most frightening experiences associated with surgery for children is forcing them to lie down on the OR table and "smothering" them with the anesthesia mask while putting them to sleep. This definitely can add to post-surgery psychological trauma for these kids. Over the years, I have found that holding children in my lap or letting them sit on the OR table to go to sleep makes for a very pleasant experience for them. I even encourage kids to go to sleep in a wagon or a car if they so choose. This can be done very easily and safely. All it takes is patience and possibly a little creativity on the part of the anesthesia personnel. As a parent, you have a right to request this type of treatment for your child. You certainly have the right to respectfully, but firmly, request that your child not be forced to lie down to be put to sleep. In fact, I will go so far as to say it is your duty to request this to help prevent trauma to your child.

F. W. Ernst, M.D. — William G. Pace III, M. D.

KEY POINT: As a parent, you are responsible for assuring that the anesthesia personnel caring for your child do their job with thoughtful, compassionate, and loving attention to its impact on the child's psyche.

Remember, too, that kids are usually much more cooperative when given a chance to participate in decisions.

When they reach the age of seven or eight, you can offer them some choices—such as deciding whether they want to "go to sleep" via an intravenous induction or a mask (or maybe even by blowing up a balloon!).

Thankfully, today's medical technology has found a way to eliminate the ghastly odor of those old-fashioned ethers! Still, it's important to remember that some anesthetic gases do carry a pungent odor. How to offset this threatening effect? Why not apply some flavored cooking oil (or even pleasingly scented lip glosses) to the inside of the breathing mask? Unfortunately, that residual smell can't be eliminated completely: over the years, I've found that it usually helps to tell the child about the "yucky" smell—like dirty gym socks—that he or she might notice, while briefly wearing the mask.

A child's sense of inner security will always be an important factor in the cooperation you get from a child during a mask induction.

Another helpful approach, of course, is to emphasize the positive aspects of anesthesia and surgery, while downplaying the negatives. You can also help create a calm atmosphere by making sure the child's favorite stuffed toys or blankets are prominently on display before and after surgery.

Recognizing the importance of such positive reinforcement, most surgical facilities today give children a small, huggable bear upon admission. The toy quickly allows the child to begin associating the surgery with something pleasant. A winning strategy!

I also counsel parents to offer their children a reward on the day of surgery—perhaps a token gift or a special treat at McDonald's or Baskin-Robbins on the way home after the surgery.

Remember, too, that many children must endure more than one operation—especially those who require multiple plastic surgeries, orthopedic surgeries for trauma or congenital malformations, or repeated tubes in their ears for recurrent ear infections. It goes almost without saying that if that first surgical experience is a positive, unthreatening one, the child will be much more cooperative—and far less frightened—when it comes to future surgical procedures.

By paying careful attention to your child's fragile psyche during surgery/anesthesia, and by making sure that the professional medical personnel involved are caring, compassionate medical practitioners with a special sensitivity to kids, you can also make sure that Fred Ernst's four-year-old nightmare never comes back to haunt your beloved child.

IN SUMMARY

- Medical professionals and parents alike need to understand one vitally important thing about preparing children for surgery: these patients are not merely "small adults" who are about to undergo an operation. In fact, they require an entirely different regimen of patient-care, from admitting to departure.

- Research shows that separating children from parents before and after surgery increases stress and trauma. For that reason, medical professionals and parents should be encouraged to find ways to keep parents and children together as much as possible during the surgical experience.

F. W. Ernst, M.D. — William G. Pace III, M. D.

- Use the tools of pre-operative education (as outlined in this chapter) to prepare your little ones for surgery in the least stressful way.

- Plan a special treat or outing for the child to look forward to after surgery, in order to reduce stress as much as possible.

CHAPTER FIVE

BEAUTY FOR A FATAL PRICE

Dr. Ernst

KEY POINTS:

- **Surgery is Never a "Piece of Cake, Even When It's Only Cosmetic"**
- **What You Don't Know About the Process Can Be Quite Hazardous to Your Health!**

Later, after the disaster struck and her life had nearly been snuffed out, Marjorie Havens would remember the phone call from her sister, Edith, and the fear she'd heard in Edith's endless stream of questions...

It was Thursday night at the Havens place on Elkridge Avenue—comedy night!

For Bob and Marjorie Havens, both in their mid -50s, watching these funny movies on the VCR every Thursday night had become a delightful weekly ritual. It was all part of their exciting new life together, now that both kids were off studying at Penn State.

How often these two "empty-nesters" had looked forward to enjoying such evenings together, once Bobby and Louise were safely settled in their dorm suites at University Park, and life on the home front had calmed down a little!

Comedy night! On this particular Thursday evening in Lancaster, a pleasant town of about 50,000 located in south-central Pennsylvania, the happy couple was in the middle of yet another Steve Martin classic, *Father of the Bride II*.

As usual, Bob had whipped up a bowl of low-fat popcorn to accompany the root beer they loved to guzzle during these goofy sessions.

"Hey, I love this guy!" sang Bob, a veteran life insurance salesman who was figuring to retire in six or seven years. "Watch this, Marge!"

He pointed to the television where Martin, playing the usual neurotic's role for which he is famous, had just discovered that his wife and his daughter were both expecting babies! In a moment, Bob and Marge were roaring together, as the pathetic Martin struggled to absorb the shocking information.

At that moment the telephone rang.

It was Edith, Marge's sister, in Grand Rapids.

"Oh . . . hi there, Edith!"

"Hello, Marge. I just called to check on you. . . All set for that surgery tomorrow?"

"Oh, sure," chuckled Marge, who still had one eye on the screen. "It's just a routine lipectomy, Edith. No big deal! Heck, I'm not even staying overnight."

"Really?" Edith sounded a little unsure. "But it's still what they call major surgery, isn't it? I mean, don't they put you under?"

"Yeah, I guess so. But, hey, the whole thing only takes about an hour. No sweat! Stop worrying, Edith—you're such a worrywart!"

There was a pause on the line; then Edith hurried on with her lecture. "Did you explain to all the doctors that you just had a tummy-tuck three months ago, when they did that hysterectomy on you?"

Marge shook her head impatiently. "Of course I explained it, Edith! My GYN guy called the weight clinic where I go. . . He must've spent half an hour on the phone with the surgeon who's doing the lipo! Stop worrying, will you?"

"Sorry, Marge. It's just that you're my little sister—you know I gotta take care of you."

"Uh-huh. All right. No problems, Sis." But Marge was hardly listening; by now her gaze had returned to the TV-set, where Woody Allen was battling a runaway fire extinguisher.

"Promise me you'll review the entire process, step by step, with the doctors—before they put you under? And make them admit Bob into the recovery room, so he can be with you? Will you do it, Marge?"

"Okay, okay . . . dammit, Edith!"

"I love you, Marge."

"Good night, Edith."

Finally, she managed to hang up. "That sister of mine," groaned Marge as she fell back on the sofa and reached for the popcorn bowl. "She's a good old gal . . . but, Lord, what a worrier!"

****

The next morning, June 14, 1991, Edith Blount's "irrational" fears about the scheduled suction lipectomy of fatty tissue from her 55-year-old sister's thighs and hips turned out to be nightmarishly justified.

Although Marge Havens and her husband Bob could not have predicted it at the time, the two of them were about to endure a desperate, edge-of-the-cliff struggle to keep Marjorie alive, after what should have been a perfectly safe "cosmetic surgery procedure" suddenly exploded into a medical crisis.

That crisis began innocuously enough, with Marge breezing through Out-Patient Admissions at Lancaster Valley General Hospital, where her cosmetic surgeon from the weight clinic performed all of his lipectomies under a long-standing arrangement. After taking some required lab tests and signing a release form authorizing the procedure, Marge received a general anesthetic intravenously, and dropped off into peaceful sleep.

Immediately, the cosmetic surgeon went to work on the suction lipectomy of fatty tissue along her hips and thighs.

Incredibly enough, however, he somehow failed to realize that with each milliliter of tissue he removed, his inert patient was actually drifting closer and closer to cardiac arrest, and possible death!

To understand how Marge's "harmless cosmetic surgery" could actually turn out to be life-threatening, let's step back for a moment and take a look at one of the potentially hazardous side-effects of the suction-lipectomy process—a condition known as "decreased blood volume."

During suction-lipectomies, two different factors trigger this sudden drop in the volume of the patient's blood. First, the body's tissues are placed under a great deal of stress during a lipectomy; the sudden cutting away of fat leaves the area in a condition not very different from the aftermath of a bad burn. The body always responds to such trauma in the same way—with the circulatory system releasing fluid to the damaged tissues, a process called "edema."

Obviously, the loss of these fluids contributes heavily to an unavoidable decline in blood volume.

At the same time, however, substantial amounts of blood are being removed from the patient's system, along with the fatty tissue excised by the surgeon. Add this blood loss to the fluid that escapes through edema, and you can end up with "hypovolemia," which is simply the medical term for decreased blood volume.

When this hypovolemia reaches a level of 20 to 25 percent of total blood volume, the patient faces a very real risk of circulatory shutdown and potentially lethal shock.

To protect against that hazard, any well-run surgical operation will keep plenty of intravenous fluids going into the patient, and will also maintain a nearby blood supply, in case of emergency.

THIS IS A KEY POINT:

If your surgeon is about to remove significant amounts of fatty tissue from your abdomen, hips, or thighs, make certain that everything necessary for the administration of blood is readily available during the procedure.

In most lipectomy procedures, of course, the amount of blood loss remains far below the danger point, and the patient sails through the operation without adverse effects.

But that wasn't the case with Marge Havens—because of a physical complication that should have raised a bright-red flag in the surgeon's office the moment she walked through the door.

In fact, Marge's past medical history was extremely significant, since she had undergone an abdominal hysterectomy—accompanied by a cosmetic "tummy tuck"—only three months prior to the procedure she was now undergoing. And that previous surgery would loom large during the next few hours because of its impact in reducing the hemoglobin level of her circulatory system.

When hypovolemia sets in, the great danger is that the iron-and-oxygen carrying protein in the blood stream, the hemoglobin, will decline to the point that the body becomes starved for oxygen, triggering shock and circulatory shutdown.

When Marge checked into Lancaster General that morning, her hemoglobin level stood at 10.5 grams, which meant that it barely surpassed the minimum standard 10.0 required for any elective surgery. In short, her hemoglobin was already at a low level—a fact which should have sent up yet another red flag for that attending surgeon and anesthesiologist.

However, neither allowed for this complication, even though he had to have known that Marge possessed only minimal hemoglobin-reserve to cover any additional blood loss. The surgeon should have calculated that a lipectomy patient will lose 1.5 grams of hemoglobin for every 500 milliliters of blood lost. Since blood loss during this procedure usually amounts to about one-third of the fatty tissue removed, the potential for threatening inroads on hemoglobin becomes very real if levels are already low.

In the case of Marge Havens, you didn't have to be a world-class mathematician to understand that, if the surgeon removed 2,000 milliliters of tissue, her hemoglobin level might very well drop to 8.5 grams—well below the danger point.

Nonetheless, the apparently unthinking surgeon proceeded with her suction-lipectomy.

Imagine his discomfort two hours later, when the medical staff in the recovery room informed him that the patient had fallen behind discharge-schedule—her vital signs had not yet stabilized. What had gone wrong here? Gradually, however, she did seem to come around, and by late afternoon she was sitting up in bed, weak and tired but otherwise okay.

And that's when the surgeon and the other medical professionals on the scene made their next mistake. Instead of remaining watchful and cautious, given her problems in recovery, they caved in to her pleading and agreed to discharge her.

Around 5 p.m., Bob Havens arrived to drive his wife home from the "harmless surgery."

Gently, he helped her into the family's green-painted Buick Skylark, and then began the 25-minute drive back to Elkridge Avenue.

It was to be a drive he would never forget.

To this day, Bob remembers how it began to rain the moment they climbed into the car. He remembers asking her about the surgery, and how she was in the middle of telling him, "I got so woozy, later, and everything kept turning black. Felt like I was fainting, really, over and over again. The strangest damn thing—"

She trailed off slowly.

Bob looked over at her.

To this day, he remembers how her broad, friendly face appeared to "freeze" on him . . . how she suddenly began to wheeze and choke. "Marge, what is it? Honey? What the hell?"

To this day, he remembers how he whipped the car into a parking lot on Winona Avenue. How he took her face in his hands—it was a mass of ugly purple blotches by then, and her eyes had rolled back in her head—and stared with horror at her sagging mouth, her lightless eyes. . .

Frantic, he skidded the car through a U-turn in the parking lot, and thundered back down Winona toward the emergency room of the hospital he and Marge had just left!

Within a matter of minutes, the ER staffers understood what they were dealing with: a major convulsive seizure, potentially lethal, triggered by decreased blood volume. In a flash, they were wheeling her toward Intensive Care—and toward a three-hour battle to keep her alive.

In the end, Marge Havens survived, mainly because she'd been very, very fortunate: she hadn't vomited and aspirated during her seizure, which meant that she'd been able to keep enough oxygen in her lungs to stay alive until the intensive care crew could begin working on her.

Three years later, Marge and Bob Havens would win a large malpractice settlement against both the cosmetic surgeon and the hospital where the procedure had been performed. But the money would never erase the horror that had visited Bob or relieve Marge of her permanent shuddering anxiety at the mere thought of hospitals and surgery.

F. W. Ernst, M.D. — William G. Pace III, M. D.

****

Rx: Plan all aspects of anesthesia well in advance

These days, of course, the popularity of cosmetic surgery has never been higher. Some of this increased fascination with "tummy tucks," "face lifts," and liposuction is the result of new technology, and some is the result of the increased emphasis on looking young and beautiful by the American public.

Today, cosmetic surgery, as opposed to reconstructive plastic surgery, is rarely performed in a hospital setting. This is both good and bad. The bad is that hospitals are the last bastion of surgical credentialing. Once out from under the protective umbrella of the hospital staff and quality control/peer review processes, there are almost no checks and balances on a surgeon's credentials. This is why it is so important for the educated plastic-surgery consumer to ask his/her cosmetic surgeon if he/she is credentialed to perform the surgery recommended at a local hospital or ambulatory surgery center.

Many of these cosmetic surgical procedures are performed with infiltration of local anesthesia, and possibly with varying degrees of intravenous sedation. Other procedures call for general anesthesia. And this is the first area of concern for any patient, who must understand one key principle about the process from the beginning:

The type of anesthesia you receive should dictate not only the medical personnel who will participate in your operation, but also the location of surgery.

Obviously, general anesthesia carries the greatest risks, and thus requires the most experienced and competent medical personnel available. There's no question that your anesthetic needs are best served by an Anesthesiologist and/or a Certified Registered Nurse Anesthetist (CRNA).

Strong consideration should also be given that the setting for the administration of any general anesthetic be either a hospital environment or an ambulatory surgery center. Of course, all accredited facilities will have the capability of handling any surgical or anesthetic complications, including the most serious: cardiac arrest.

In addition, all free-standing or independent ambulatory surgery centers and doctors' offices should have a policy and procedure in place for direct admission to a local hospital—preferably less than 10 miles away—if a complication should arise.

Note well: This is an important point about which you, the patient, should always inquire.

You need to have absolute assurance that, should a complication arise, you can be transferred directly to a hospital setting. Additionally, you might inquire about the percentage of patients who have required such hospital admission in the past. (A one-to-two percent admission rate is generally considered acceptable; higher rates should alert you to possible problems with the surgical center.)

Another important point: although local anesthesia with sedation does not carry the same degree of risk as general anesthesia, it is by no means an "innocuous procedure." Often this type of anesthesia will be administered right in the surgeon's office. Because sedation can lead to differing degrees of patient consciousness, requiring careful attention to the management of airways, you need to be assured that a competent health-care provider will be in attendance at all times to monitor your vital signs and to manage your airway, should that become necessary.

Such tasks are best accomplished by staff certified in anesthesia. A pulse oximeter, which is an instrument designed to measure your blood oxygen saturation, is also considered a required monitoring device these days. But you also need a health-care provider who is knowledgeable about the data it provides, and who can take whatever steps might be required to ensure your safety. Make certain that these services are available in your surgeon's office, and don't forget that all drugs used for sedation can lower respiration and thus can lower oxygen saturation. Indeed, if it's not monitored properly, heavy sedation can cause respiratory arrest, which can even produce cardiac arrest in extreme cases.

When it comes to the business of suction lipectomy, the single most commonly performed cosmetic operation worldwide, we can learn a great deal from the very unfortunate case of Marge Havens.

Lesson number one should be:

During your initial conference with the surgeon, determine exactly how much tissue is to be removed—and then be careful to determine the amount of blood loss (and hemoglobin depletion) that you can expect.

As it has been known and taught since the early 1980s, liposuction as a sole procedure has a mortality rate barely measurable. Almost all complications associated with liposuction are related to one issue—VOLUME.

If your surgeon is planning to remove a significant amount of tissue, insist that the facility provide everything required for the successful administration of blood, just in case your hemoglobin level becomes suspect during the operation. Remember that many free-standing ambulatory surgery centers and doctors' offices do not have this capability, which should make you question whether or not you really wish to be operated on at one of them.

You should discuss tissue-removal amounts with your surgeon, while also reviewing the standard guidelines in your state for the top limits of tissue that can be removed on any given day. Many states have legislated volume amount limits for outpatient surgery centers and doctors' offices. These volume limits range from a low of 3000 ml to a top of 5000 ml in some states. Clearly, some disagreement exists regarding upper limits for safety. Furthermore, the larger the amount removed, the greater are the projected risks.

Universally, the poor results with liposuction are a result of combining multiple procedures under one anesthetic. This assumes that one very long procedure (longer than six hours) is safer than two shorter procedures (less than three hours each) separated by a month or so.

According to Dr. Paul Howard, a prominent Birmingham, AL plastic surgeon, "Plastic surgeons by training and nature are innovators who desperately want to please our patients. But, like a good parent, we must learn the limits of what we do, define how much, how long, and where we do it, and consistently stick to our guns by saying no to our children (patients). Sometimes, this can be difficult to achieve."

It's important to remember that getting careless about blood levels in cosmetic surgery can produce some horrific results.

In another ghastly example of what can go wrong in this type of supposedly "harmless" surgery, a 53-year-old female patient visited a free-standing surgery center for a scheduled face-lift and surgery of the upper and lower eyelids. But her medical history included a lengthy bout with anemia, the cause of which had never been completely investigated by her family physician.

During a check of her pre-operative hemoglobin on the day of surgery, the level was found to be 8.5 grams. Because the levels were too low for safety, this elective surgery was canceled.

Of course, hospitals, surgeons, and patients don't respond very well to cancellations on the day of surgery! Hoping to make things right, the surgeon called for further blood tests to determine the cause of the anemia and then rescheduled the surgery for four days later.

Soon a partial blood work-up had been completed; it showed some abnormalities that needed further scrutiny. Once again the surgery was cancelled, this time by the medical director of the facility.

Amazingly, however, the surgeon elected to perform the surgery in his office—and without further tests.

Fortunately, no major complications ensued in this case. Yet it remains disturbingly true that, if the proper pre-operative hemoglobin test had been ordered by the surgeon's office well in advance of the surgery, the cancellation and inconvenience could have been avoided.

Another frequent cosmetic procedure is breast augmentation. This procedure frequently takes place in a surgeon's office, and under local anesthesia and sedation. One key area of concern here is the amount of local anesthetic to be injected, since large amounts are frequently utilized in order to keep the patient quiet on the operating table.

The danger in using such large doses is obvious: too much anesthetic can produce toxic reactions, resulting is seizures and perhaps even respiratory and cardiac arrest.

Unfortunately, not every physician who uses local anesthetics has a clear understanding of the safe-dosage range for all of the varieties employed. Nor do these sedative-wielding surgeons always know enough about the two different chemical classes to which the anesthetics belong. Unfortunately, such lack of knowledge can lead to dangerous allergic reactions among patients, another significant danger.

KEY POINT:

Make sure to discuss the allergic-potential of using local anesthetics in your operation with your surgeon and his anesthesia personnel, long before surgery day!

There's no denying that cosmetic surgery patients **do** face significant risks. And yet we as a society continue to embrace these procedures in our never-ending quest for youthful beauty. We are certainly not recommending to you that cosmetic surgery is inadvisable because, most of the time, procedures such as tummy tucks, face-lifts, and liposuction occur without a hitch, vastly improving the lives of the patients who undergo them.

But in order to make certain that your surgery does not become one of the dangerous exceptions, you need to follow the instructions we have just reviewed. After that, we wish you a happy surgery!

IN SUMMARY

- Remember that surgery is never a "piece of cake," even when it's "only cosmetic"; you must take the same careful precautions about choosing a good surgeon and a good anesthesia team that you would take for any other kind of surgery.
- The type of anesthesia you receive should dictate not only the anesthesia personnel who will participate in your surgery, but also the location in which the procedure will take place.
- If you are planning to have a significant amount of tissue removed via suction lipectomy, make certain that the anesthesia team is fully equipped to administer blood, should that need arise.
- Remember that local anesthesia also carries some hazards (as outlined in this chapter); do not take it for granted!

F. W. Ernst, M.D. — William G. Pace III, M. D.

Truth, Lies and the OR

CHAPTER SIX

FOREIGN MEDICAL GRADUATES

Dr. Pace

KEY POINT:

- **While there are many outstanding health professionals from foreign countries now at work in the United States, surgery/anesthesia patients should be extremely vigilant when consulting foreign doctors: the blunt fact is that some of them have been inadequately prepared for careers in medicine at non-board-certified, second-rate medical schools.**

For 37-year-old Patty Killebrew of Enid, Oklahoma, the tragedy would begin on a rainy Tuesday night in the mid 1990s, as she watched a beautiful woman named Julia Roberts walk gracefully across her TV screen.

The movie was *Pretty Woman,* and this was at least the third time that Patty had watched it. Patty was alone again tonight.

Her 10-year marriage to Clint Killebrew, the night manager at the South Enid Harvest Fresh Super Market, had exploded into an ugly divorce only eight months earlier. Deeply wounded by what she regarded as Clint's betrayal, Patty was struggling through the worst depression of her life.

Night after night, she'd been trying to fill the void in her life with food—jumbo-sized bags of potato chips, sugary doughnuts, and quart-sized containers of fudge ripple ice cream.

What a bummer! Patty knew that all these calories were an effort to compensate for the painful loss of her husband. She was also deeply alarmed at her weight gain—four and five pounds a month. All her life, it seemed she'd been struggling to prevent the onset of what she jokingly described as "the ultimate Fat Attack—I'm afraid I'm gonna end up looking like the Goodyear Blimp!"

And now her worst fears were being realized.

Only five feet, two inches tall, the unhappy bank teller, was already up to 170 pounds! Of course, she'd always been rather "chunky" (that was the word she preferred to use, instead of "fat"). She'd grown up hating the sound of the nickname, "Fatty Patty!", that some of the crueler kids at Markle Middle School had given her. . .

A blimp!

Yes, she needed to get this problem under control. And yet the mere thought of beginning an exercise program and getting serious about her runaway carbohydrate-intake made Patty's heart sink. Maybe tomorrow she'd start shaping up . . . maybe go to see that nutritionist that Bev down at the bank had been recommending. But right now, tonight, she felt so miserable—all she wanted was another bowl of fudge ripple ice cream!

She sighed, and reached for the cellophane bag of chips.

Sitting in the twilight in her tiny apartment, she watched the actress whom *People* magazine had named "One of the World's Ten Most Beautiful Women" flirt coyly with the incredibly handsome Richard Gere.

Life just wasn't fair.

That slim, svelte Julia Roberts probably ate all the ice cream she wanted and never gained a pound.

Well, there was no cure for it . . . or was there?

As the movie ended and the credits began rolling across the screen, Patty was reaching for her green handbag, then flipping open the tiny silver dolphin that served as its clasp.

Yes, the article she'd clipped a week ago was still inside. Now she pulled the ragged piece of newsprint out of its hiding place, unfolded it, smoothed it in her lap and read the headline for at least the tenth time in recent days:

BAYVIEW SURGEON CLAIMS "AMAZING" LOSS
POSSIBLE THROUGH USE OF DARING NEW
STOMACH "STAPLING" TECHNIQUE

Rather breathlessly, the article went on to describe a "marvelous new breakthrough" in controlling obesity . . . some kind of experimental new surgical technique in which the surgeon implanted surgical staples across the length of the stomach in order to inhibit digestion and thus prevent calories from being absorbed into the bloodstream by the small intestine.

Did it work? According to the surgeon, an "upbeat and enthusiastic" young doctor from Saudi Arabia whom the article named as Dr. Falud Kashabi, this daring new method of shutting down the body's digestive system in order to trigger weight-loss was a "gift from heaven."

And there was more: Dr. Kashabi could virtually "guarantee" the results! Although he'd only arrived in this country a few months before, he had participated in a similar program in his native land—and had watched a number of obese patients shed 50, even 60 pounds within a year of undergoing the "staple-surgery" procedure!

Should Patty call this enterprising young doctor at the Willard Weight Clinic and find out more about his new technique? Maybe . . . She sat there, staring at the news clipping, and once again the willow-slim image of Julia Roberts rose before her, the luckiest woman on earth!

So be it. She would call his clinic, first thing in the morning.

The medical scenario that followed was as infuriatingly irresponsible as it was tragic.

Dr. Kashabi, as it turned out, had never performed a single "stomach-stapling" procedure on his own—although he had watched two or three of the experimental operations performed at his brother-in-law's Weight-Loss Clinic in Riyadh.

Nonetheless, as he testified later at his multi-million dollar malpractice trial in Oklahoma City, he felt no compunctions about assuring Patty Killbrew that he could help her shed 50-60 pounds with his dubious staples.

He also showed her a few "before-and -after" photos that were simply generic photos of people who had managed to lose weight—photos that had in fact been obtained from the medical section of the local public library!

Tragically, Patty herself was still so distraught over her failed marriage and her eating disorder that she failed to scrutinize the doctor's credentials, or even to ask detailed questions about the nature of the "stapling" procedure.

Patty Killebrew became a classic example of how a lack of knowledge about impending surgery can actually endanger your life; in the end, she based her decision to proceed with the operation almost entirely on the strength of the newspaper story that had caught her eye.

Three years later, reviewing the file, I positively writhed in my chair as I listened to the horror story that had ensued after the insertion of the staples in poor Patty's stomach.

Although the 45-minute procedure itself appeared to have gone smoothly enough, there were signs even before Patty left the recovery room that something was amiss; she was vomiting continuously, and quite painfully.

Dr. Kashabi shrugged—what was a little vomiting after all?--and sent her home.

The next day, when the nausea had not lessened and Patty finally found the strength to call the doctor about it, his nurse simply prescribed narcotics.

Unfortunately, they didn't help.

But when Patty dialed Dr. Kashabi's office the next day, she received an unpleasant shock: nobody answered the phone, all day long. On the third day, feeling terribly ill, she finally checked herself into an emergency room.

Maddeningly, the ER physician refused to examine her, because she was the surgeon's patient! Instead, he called Dr. Kashabi . . . who quickly recommended more narcotics. Once again, however, poor Patty was overwhelmed by her pain, and checked into a second ER. And once again, the ER medical staff refused to examine another doctor's patient.

When the staffers at the second emergency room called the doctor, he simply told them, "Oh, she's already been treated!" Once again, the suffering woman was dispatched to her home.

On the following day, she was so ill that an ambulance had to be summoned.

And this time, when the attendants finally brought her into the ER on a stretcher, Patty Killebrew was dead.

Indeed, a later autopsy showed that the young woman had ruptured her entire staple line, allowing everything she ate to seep into the peritoneum, so that she died of acute peritonitis.

Reviewing the file in this brutal case of malpractice, I was hardly surprised to discover that three additional malpractice actions had already been launched against this same physician.

The second travesty of good medical practice was similar to the first, except that the patient was a male who ruptured his stomach in the recovery room, and then died on the way back to the operating room—even as he was being watched by the medical staff!

The third horror involved a 75-year-old woman who suffered from minimal diverticulitis of the colon, with a nearly normal white blood count and minimal findings. In her case, a barium enema showed some narrowing of the colon (certainly not enough to warrant surgery), along with fecal masses scattered throughout the same organ. The doctor responded to this finding by giving the patient one capsule of neomycin, a drug often used for sterilization of the colon.

He then proceeded to operate and do a resection of the diseased portion of the colon, along with a reconnection of the colon to itself—even though the fecal material was present! This operation was doomed to failure, as you might expect. A terrible post-operative infection set in almost immediately and necessitated a permanent colostomy from which the poor lady would suffer for the rest of her life.

In the end, this was the only one of four cases against Dr. Kashabi that actually went to trial—where the foreign physician promptly told the jury that neomycin can sterilize feces and that proper bowel preparation is not necessary before surgery! He lost the case, and rightfully so.

The fourth case against this surgical charlatan was one in which he treated an obese gentleman who did have some diverticulitis, but who certainly did not require surgery. Apparently having learned by now that "bowel preparation" is indeed necessary, the scalpel-waving Dr. Kashabi at least attempted some superficial preparation.

Unfortunately, he also elected to remove the man's appendix in the middle of the surgery—a completely unnecessary bit of bungling that is definitely contraindicated when performing a resection of the colon. (There's a significant risk that the appendiceal stump may "blow out" in such a scenario, producing lethal peritonitis, which is precisely what happened in this case.)

As you might expect, there was massive contamination of the peritoneum on the second operation, and so the desperate surgeon removed all of the patient's colon and connected his small intestine directly to the rectum—thereby condemning his patient to a grim regimen of several diarrhea attacks daily for the rest of his life.

I assumed that the State Medical Board would act quickly to bar this surgeon from practice. However, I was wrong: the Board ruled that the surgeon would be restricted to hand surgery—which calls for some of the most critical and demanding skills in the entire field of surgery!

****

Rx: Keep an Open Mind About Foreign Medical Graduates, but Remember to Remain Vigilant, Since Many Have not Been Adequately Prepared to Perform Surgery

Like many other practicing physicians in the United States who were trained in foreign countries, Dr. Kashabi lacked the rigorous preparation that is absolutely essential for successful surgery.

And let me be quite clear about this: there are many foreign-trained doctors who perform outstanding service as top-quality physicians with scrupulous dedication to the highest standards of the medical profession. However, common sense also tells you that you must remain vigilant about undergoing surgery from foreign doctors, some of whom have not been taught to meet these same high standards in their countries of origin.

Another foreign-trained doctor devised his own combination of operations in order to make obese people thin "overnight." By the time his unethical practice came to my attention, he had done so many expensive procedures that he was able to build an auditorium in which to lecture and recruit patients!

This highly unethical doctor charged $4,000 in the 1990s for his "fat operation" and then added $1,500 to remove the patient's gallbladder—which he routinely accomplished, whether the organ was diseased or not. He had performed thousands of these procedures by the time I was called in to review a malpractice action in which a former patient charged that he had required her to undergo a second surgery to enlarge her stomach opening—after her endless vomiting and agony had caused her to lose more than 100 pounds.

In addition to expanding the opening by one millimeter (about 1/32nd of an inch), he removed her entirely normal gallbladder—which he'd forgotten the first time around! After that second operation, when the surgeon found her wandering in a hallway, dazed and dizzy, he ordered "stat" (emergency) blood chemical determinations, but nobody checked them—or at least not until she was found dead in her bed, two hours later.

The surgeon fought this case of blatant malpractice all the way to the courthouse steps ... and then settled. The plaintiff's lawyer later informed me, "off the record," that this surgeon had settled 28 straight malpractice cases before that—he had never once been to court! The surgeon continues to practice even today.

Generalizations are always dangerous, of course, but it's revealing that both of these defendants were foreign medical school graduates, and that both spoke English with accents that were extremely difficult to penetrate.

Whenever I have described the potential dangers of undergoing surgery performed by foreign-trained physicians, I receive buckets of hate mail and phone calls—and that's precisely what happened after I wrote an article on this subject for the *Bulletin of the American College of Surgeons* in 1994. In that article, I pointed out that the majority of the malpractice problems I had encountered had involved non-board-certified, foreign medical graduates. I was simply relating my experience, without exaggerating. One angry caller insisted that I call the foreign doctors by a special term: "International Medical Doctors," or IMD.

As politely as I could, however, I maintained my position, and continued to point out that since medical schools in the United States are the best in the world, without question, these foreign physicians will remain "Foreign Medical Graduates," or "FMG," in any references I may make to them.

In my opinion, graduates of foreign medical schools can take three steps to improve perception of their professionalism in the United States. They can:

- Obtain board certification in this country;
- Improve communication skills in English;
- Adhere to high ethical standards of practice.

IN SUMMARY

- While there are many outstanding health professionals from foreign countries now at work in the United States, surgery/anesthesia patients should be extremely vigilant when consulting foreign doctors: the blunt fact is that some of them have been inadequately prepared for careers in medicine at non-board-certified, second-rate medical schools.

- One extremely risky procedure that is sometimes offered to the public by foreign-trained surgeons involves "experimental" treatments for obesity. Don't be tempted!.

F. W. Ernst, M.D. — William G. Pace III, M. D.

CHAPTER SEVEN

'DOC IN A BOX'

Dr. Ernst

KEY POINT:

- **"Drive-By" Medicine May Be More Convenient, but it's a Serious Mistake to Sacrifice Quality Medical Care for Mere Convenience.**

Every once in a while, a patient or a friend of mine will turn to me and ask, "Dr. Fred, what's your opinion of those drive-by medical clinics that have been popping up all over the country?"

Of course, my response is always the same.

"Got a minute?" I ask my interrogator. "Can I buy you a cup of coffee?"

"Why, sure . . ."

Once we're settled in, with our feet up and the java steaming in our cups, I tell my friend the story of Ivy Zebulon Crockett, one of the best outside jump-shooters I ever watched play basketball. . .

****

Saturday night fever!

Ivy Crockett, the outside shooting threat, was the first man to go to his knees.

He closed his eyes. He folded his hands and took a few deep breaths. While his teammates fell into position around him, he was already praying silently: *Dear Lord, help me tonight. I don't ask you for a win—that wouldn't be right. All I'm askin' is, keep me out of harm's way!*

The others were also praying by now. Hands folded, they were looking up at Coach Barlow. Waiting. Each man was feeling the tension; each man was doing his best to come to terms with his own fear. "O Lord," intoned the veteran coach, as his eyes swept the circle of 14 young players, "help us to perform tonight in a way that will bring glory to your name. . . "

It was Saturday night at the Hotchkiss Arena on the outskirts of Birmingham, and for the 14 young men in the green-and-gold Willowbrook Community College uniforms, destiny had finally arrived. If they could just win one more ballgame—just find a way, somehow, to defeat their mighty cross-town rivals, the Jaguars of Jackson Heights College!--these excited young ballplayers would be bringing home the first-ever conference trophy to Willowbrook.

What were they doing in this vast, echoing arena, anyway?

For the past two years, these 14 hotshots had been playing their games in a scuffed, drafty gymnasium where nails stuck up from some of the bleachers and the warped baskets sent balls caroming off into the crowd as if they'd been launched from giant slingshots.

But not now. Not tonight.

Because this year, against all the odds, the Crusaders of Willowbrook had put together a once-in-a-lifetime season. Somehow, they'd managed to win five straight nail-biters in overtime . . . and had then gone on to upset powerhouse Riverview Community College in the season finale.

They didn't belong here. But here they were, in the 12,000-seat Hotchkiss Arena, with a legitimate chance to nail down a conference title in a ballgame that none of them would ever forget. "O Lord," prayed the soft-spoken, silver-haired Barlow, as he walked slowly around the circle of kneeling athletes, "Let each one of us find tonight the thing he needs most—as a student, as an athlete—and let our play further glorify our Heavenly Father!"

He paused, and every eye turned toward him.

"Men," said Rex Barlow, grinning at them like they were his own kids, "I'm so proud of you I could bust. . .

"—Go get 'em!"

Now they rose as one man; as one man they turned and headed for the big swinging doors that led from the dressing room out to the tunnel.

Loping along the runway, and still breathing deep, Ivy Z. Crockett began to rehearse all of the things he would have to do on this night, if his team were to have even an outside shot at winning. . .

First, he'd have to keep his cool against the Jaguar full-court press: those guys could just plain bring it, and if you forgot about the passing lanes and the "curl-back" moves in your haste to bring the ball up the floor, those hawk-eyed scrappers would eat you for lunch.

Next, he'd have to keep repeating the magical phrase that had been carrying him through the last 17 games: "Arch and release!" For Ivy Crockett, a physically gifted 20-year-old from the St. Xavier Housing Complex over on the east side of the city, basketball was more than a sport: it was virtually a religion. And like any religious devotee, he had worked out a series of rituals and prayers over the years.

If you watched this rangy, 6-foot-5 point guard in the bright blue sneakers zoom skyward to launch his jumper—watched really closely—you'd see his lips moving just as he let go of the ball: "Arch and release!" It was a simple prescription for success, designed to remind Ivy of the two key ingredients required for any accurate shot: plenty of "arch" on the ball, as it whistled toward the distant basket, and plenty of follow-through from his shooting arm and shoulder, so that the delivery would be smooth and consistent, every single time.

Arch and release! When the tip-off came, at seven minutes past eight, Ivy was already muttering the phrase to himself again and again. Would this be his night? Maybe so . . . Like magic, the tipped ball caromed off an opposing player's shoulder and into Ivy's hands. And then he was off. He was a blur, coming down the right side of the court. . . Like a crazed water bug on the surface of a motionless pond, Ivy Crockett was skitterring across the top of the key, juking to the left, dribbling the ball between his legs, finding an open space near the foul line. Then he was airborne, hanging motionless in space for a moment, as if actually defying gravity.

Arch and release.

Sweet as a candy-colored, summer rainbow, the basketball soared through a perfect parabola—then hissed through the net!

A moment later, you could hear the vast throng out in the arena chanting the same two syllables over and over again: "I-VY! I-VY!"

And so it began—a bruising, two-hour struggle in which the out-manned Crusaders fought desperately to stave off the superior firepower of the Jaguar scoring machine. Armed with the best small-college center in the state (a six-ten titan with arms of hammered iron) and two brutally powerful forwards, the Jaguars would out-muscle the Crusaders around the basket all night long.

But again and again, it was Ivy Crockett who would bring them back—while nailing seven straight three-pointers early in the second half, and making one steal after another in the final stages of the game.

Somehow, the Willowbrook kids had managed to stay close enough to have a chance.

With 14 seconds left on the clock, they trailed by one.

But they had the ball. Better yet, Ivy had the ball, was dribbling it slowly across the time-line, with one eye on the huge, overhead game-clock, and another on his frantic teammates, all of whom seemed to be racing back and forth beneath the enemy basket, while hollering furiously for the ball.

But Crockett knew what he had to do.

First the electrifying "crossover dribble"—the move that he had worked on so many times in practice—which left the man guarding him flat-footed, faked right out of the play. Then the drive from the top of the key, down the lane, with the entire Jaguar defense collapsing on him.

"SIX . . . FIVE . . . FOUR!"

Then the "pull-up." Another cat-quick move from the Crockett bag of tricks, and then the leap into the jump-shot.

"THREE . . . TWO!"

Arch and release!

The ball was still in the air when the game-ending buzzer went off—but Ivy Crockett never saw it rip through the net.

No. At the moment the ball went into the hoop and the crowd came roaring up to celebrate the Crusader upset of the Jaguars, Ivy Crockett was crashing onto the hardwood floor.

Landing, after that mighty jumper, he'd stepped on another player's foot. And now he was down, flat on his back, writhing in agony and clutching his right hand, which had been caught beneath him when he lost his balance and slammed into the floorboards.

A moment later, Coach Barlow was bending above him.

The championship was forgotten for a few minutes, while the coach demanded, "Wiggle your fingers!" and "Flap your wrist!"

But Ivy couldn't. His whole hand felt numb.

"Coach . . . I think I mighta broken a bone. Remember two years ago, when I broke one in the other hand? It feels exactly the same!"

Coach Barlow put an arm around him. "Get showered up, Ivy, and I'll run you over to the Wilmer Clinic, myself."

Because Willowbrook Community College was so small, with only 600 students, its teams were required to play without the services of a regular doctor. And so the sprained knees and pulled groins and occasional broken bones all ended up at the same place: the Wilmer Clinic, over on 32nd Street, one of those "free-standing" medical clinics in which "drive-by" patients without appointments could simply "drop in" to consult with the part-time doctors.

But Ivy Crockett was hurting, and he didn't have any choice.

He was about to pay a deeply unsettling visit to what the medical profession calls "A Doc In A Box". . .

****

Rx: Watch Out For The Hazards of "Drive-By-Medicine"

The type of "free-standing" medical clinic that would treat Ivy Crockett is part of a very interesting—and disturbing— trend in medicine: the proliferation of "drive-by" treatment centers. These hastily erected medical facilities first started popping up 20 to 30 years ago, as an alternative to the high-priced "acute care" then available in hospital emergency rooms, where lengthy waits for service were quite common.

The "drive-by" sites soon caught on, and during the next decade or so, they began to expand their "acute services" into primary care. Once again, the selling-point was simple enough: the "drive-by" offered a quick alternative to the endless delays that were frequently encountered "at the doctor's office."

Soon various other kinds of specialized clinics were springing up like mushrooms on the medical landscape; some dealt exclusively in workmen's compensation injuries, for example, while others focused on pediatrics or mental health or other kinds of medical services.

It goes without saying, of course, that these kinds of clinic settings do offer some advantages in terms of speed and economy. But there are also some very serious drawbacks, starting with the fact that some of the physicians in these clinics may not be board-certified in some area of medicine, including, especially, family practice and emergency medicine.

It's also true that some of the doctors practicing in these "drive-bys" will be international medical graduates who have received some—maybe even all—of their medical training outside the continental United States. You'll also find that a number of these facilities are accredited only at the state health board level, and that the standards and guidelines for this type of accreditation vary greatly from one state to the next.

It's also important to note that not all of these kinds of facilities hold accreditation from the highest level available in this country, which is certification from the Joint Commission on Accreditation of Healthcare Organizations (JCAHO).

But what do all of these reservations and qualifications actually mean to you, the consumer of health care?

Well, for starters, you should understand that you may well run the risk of receiving less-than-optimum medical care in these kinds of facilities. That is especially true in any situation where your health needs might better be served by a medical specialist than by a "primary care" physician.

For example: Did you know that a simple facial laceration can escalate into a major cosmetic nightmare if the original treatment is not provided by a physician completely knowledgeable in cosmetic repair? Such expertise must include the use of the correct type of suture material and the correct timing for removal of stitches, if the doctor hopes to minimize permanent scarring.

Another good example concerns treatment of injuries over joint areas or at sites that involve tendons and nerves. Such lacerations—along with trauma, in many cases—to tendons and nerves, if unrecognized and untreated, can easily result in decrease in function, and even disability.

And once that impairment of function has set in, it may be too late to repair the damage and restore full function.

Another concern for "Doc In A Box" patients should be the frequent lack of backup support and follow-up service in areas such as radiology. Often these drive-by clinics don't have a radiologist on hand, which means that an expert in radiology is not available to read X-rays at the time of initial treatment. Instead, the facility will probably employ a "radiologist consultant" who may not be looking at the films for one to several days.

In some clinics, no radiologist will ever see the films, and the scrutiny of the all-important X-rays will be left entirely to the primary care physician—who usually has less experience in this highly specialized field. That's how patients sometimes walk out of these clinics with undiagnosed bone fractures.

Another problem with the free-standing clinics is their lack of secondary orthopedic care. The fact is that most primary care physicians aren't fully trained in the art of setting bone fractures and reading post-setting films to be sure the fracture has been fully realigned.

In cases of this kind, a patient's needs are best served by an orthopedic specialist. And the same can be said for cases involving athletes who sustain injuries on the field. These days, of course, the field of sports medicine has become a recognized sub-specialty of orthopedics. But not all orthopedic surgeons are well-versed and current in all the finer points of treating athletic injuries, which means that, in many cases, an injured athlete's needs may be served best by a specialist in orthopedic sports medicine.

Certainly, that's a truism for those athletes who are hoping to win college scholarships. Our professional athletes invariably receive top-level specialty-care for their injuries, as well.

Truth, Lies and the OR

But that's simply not true for many athletes on the high school and small community college level—which brings us straight back to an amazingly talented young man named Ivy Z. Crockett.

As soon as the wincing and grimacing Ivy Crockett arrived at the Wilma Clinic in Birmingham, he began to tell everybody in earshot that he'd broken his hand. "I busted a bone in the other one," he explained to the duty-nurse in the lobby, "and believe me, I know just how it feels."

But the examining physician—we'll call him Dr. Knowbetter—wasn't convinced by Ivy's diagnosis, or by his yelps and moans of pain, each time he touched the area of the injury. First Dr. Knowbetter visually examined the hand; then he ordered X-rays. But as often happens in these hurry-up clinics, the good doctor requested only two views—front to back and side to side. No oblique films were taken. This is important as some bone fractures may only show up well on an oblique X-ray.

And all too soon, young Ivy was sent on his way, with the doctor's diagnosis still ringing in his ears: "All you've got is a bad bruise!"

Wrong.

After two full weeks, the kid's hand hurt worse than ever! And that wasn't all: each time he turned it at the wrist, he could distinctly hear the "clicking" of bones abrading each other. The young man became so alarmed that he finally consulted a school chum's father—who just happened to be a medical doctor.

The M.D took one look... and quickly referred the hurting young man to an orthopedic hand specialist. And guess what? Although it was fully three weeks late, the surgeon finally arranged for all of the appropriate X-rays to be taken.

You guessed it.

Ivy's right hand was broken—and had been broken since the moment he tangled with the Jackson Heights Jaguar and hit the deck at high speed.

Quickly, the young athlete was put into an arm cast, in the hope that the bone might heal without surgery. (Had such painful surgery been required—and it seemed likely at the time—it would have necessitated the insertion of a "pin" and probably also a bone graft.)

But Ivy Crockett was lucky. Although he would spend 12 uncomfortable weeks in the cast, he did manage to heal without the surgery. Still, if his fracture had been properly diagnosed at the start, proper healing probably wouldn't have taken more than a month or so.

Of course, it's also true that if the original X-rays had been reviewed by a radiologist within 24 hours, the primary care doctor's misdiagnosis could have been corrected before it caused additional problems. But Ivy had gone to a "Doc In A Box," and, in this particular case, to a clinic that didn't bother to keep a radiologist on hand for consultations.

Too bad. But it's hardly a new story. And another example of how these drive-by clinics frequently fail to provide adequate care for athletes occurred at another facility in the Birmingham area, only a few months after Ivy Crockett's misadventure.

That second case involved trauma to the fingers of a college student who had been injured during an intramural football game. In this case, also, inadequate X-rays were ordered. After these indicated "no fractures," the complaining student was sent on his way. Yet only three weeks later, he wound up in the office of an orthopedic specialist—and quickly showed him the large "bulge" in his palm, while explaining that he was unable to flex his middle finger

The orthopedist's diagnosis was unsettling, to say the least; he quickly informed the young man that he'd ruptured the flexor tendon to his middle finger. He also pointed out that the injury was undoubtedly present at the time of the original examination by the "Doc In A Box" physician. Had the Doc only checked properly for this injury, surgery could have quickly repaired it. As it was, however, the needless delay made the operation both technically more difficult and less certain of success.

It's interesting to note that the hand is one of the most anatomically complex regions of the human body. Had our "Box Doc" known more about it—or had he taken the time to inspect this young man's hand more closely—the trauma victim might not have faced potential permanent disability of the affected hand. But the sad fact is that this drive-by facility did not offer on-the-spot consultations by a specialist in orthopedic surgery, as is usually the case in hospital emergency rooms.

Another incident occurring in California involved a teenager who sustained an injury to his index finger during a fall from a motor scooter. The victim was initially seen in a "walk-in" clinic where X-rays were obtained that showed damage to the finger. He was then referred to a plastic surgeon who was untrained in hand surgery.

The boy's finger was placed in a splint, and he was discharged without further instructions. Six weeks later, he ended up in the office of an orthopedic hand specialist, who took X-rays that showed a chronic dislocated finger.

The medical outcome was quite unfortunate: surgery offered the only possible way to correct the problem, because of the time lag that had occurred since the original injury. In the end, the teenager recovered only limited motion of the affected finger.

What important lessons can we learn about the inherent weaknesses of the "Doc In A Box" approach to health care? Furthermore, what can we learn from the increasingly frequent practice of primary care physicians rendering care in areas that are out of their expertise?

One key insight emerges immediately: there's no doubt that this country is now undergoing some major changes in the way that health care gets delivered to patients.

Perhaps the most significant change, these days, is the movement towards "managed health care," and the resulting increase in primary care physicians (along with an ever-accelerating decrease in the use of specialists).

Supposedly, this approach to health care is the answer to reducing the "spiraling costs" of contemporary medicine.

But there's a problem with this strategy: today the field of medicine is so broad and so complex that it's virtually impossible for any health-care physician to be knowledgeable in all areas.

Somehow, this vitally important fact seems to have escaped health maintenance organization executives, government officials, and others who are setting down policies for the delivery of health care in this country

And the three case histories we have just reviewed are classic examples of what can happen when primary care physicians render care in areas where they're not completely knowledgeable.

Although a more in-depth discussion of the many problems linked to managed health care is beyond the scope of this book, there's no doubt that such an inquiry is long overdue... before the American health care system collapses into the kind of chaos that will leave millions of citizens increasingly in harm's way.

IN SUMMARY

- "Drive-by" medicine may be more convenient, but it's a serious mistake to sacrifice quality medical care for mere convenience.

- Many of these free-standing medical clinics offer services by foreign-trained doctors whose training and experience may be suspect. You can't afford to take the chance!

- Along with the "drive-by" doctors, the primary care physicians now being employed by HMOs all across the country often don't have the specialized medical training to deal with your particular health problem.

F. W. Ernst, M.D. — William G. Pace III, M. D.

Truth, Lies and the OR

CHAPTER EIGHT

OFFICE –BASED SURGERY
Tragedy In Pensacola

Dr. Ernst

When the cosmetic surgery patient suddenly went into "Stage 4"—a life-threatening emergency in general anesthesia that's also known as "overdose"—nobody in the doctor's office-based surgical suite happened to notice. The 26-year-old RN (also the doctor's girlfriend) who was supposed to be monitoring the IV propofol-drip continued to pump the powerful hypnotic-sedative drug deep into the patient's brain. But that brain was already swamped with the anesthetic and was already sinking into severe medullary depression. While the daydreaming plastic surgeon proceeded with his $10,000 "chin tuck" and "breast augmentation" operation, the middle-aged woman on the table was slowly beginning to die. . . .

KEY POINT:

- Research indicates there are significantly more complications and deaths for surgeries done in office-based settings vs. ambulatory surgery centers. This disparity is even greater when comparing office-based surgeries to surgeries performed in hospitals.

It was raining again.

"My goodness—another thunderstorm!" Mildred Harbison shouted at her sister Ellie. "Shall we make a run for it?"

"You bet!" Ellie shouted back. "Try and stay under my umbrella!"

A moment later, the two of them were lurching down the front porch steps. Giggling like a couple of school girls—though both women were actually in their early 40s—they splashed their way down the sidewalk toward Ellie's silver-blue Toyota Camry.

The wind rose, turned, and whipped through the clumps of Spanish moss that dangled from the branches of the live oak tree in Ellie's front yard.

Drenched, the two of them fell into the front seat of the streaming car.

"What a mess!" exclaimed Mildred.

"That's Pensacola in August," said her sister. "Every afternoon, three o'clock, here comes the thunderstorm. It's the Gulf of Mexico – unstable air. But don't worry. We've got plenty of time."

"I'm not worried," said Mildred. "Actually, I'm kind of enjoying this whole thing. I feel like a kid again!"

Ellie grinned at her, slid the key into the ignition. The Toyota pulled slowly away from the rain-swamped curb, and the windshield wipers began their monotonous clattering.

They were headed toward the Archway Medical Center on Myrtle Grove Road.

Mildred Harbison, visiting her sister from Minneapolis, was about to undergo cosmetic surgery.

Truth, Lies and the OR

****

Ellie parked the car beneath the green awning that fronted the clinic. For a few moments, anyway, they were out of the rain.

"You're not nervous, are you?" Ellie was studying her sister carefully. After her brutally painful divorce, one year earlier, Mildred had become subdued and fretful. She'd also drifted into a major clinical depression—not uncommon, her psychiatrist had pointed out, among middle-aged women whose husbands had left them for much younger "trophy" wives. Watching the disaster from afar, Ellie had often cried to see her beloved older sister going through so much pain. "You need to put this disaster behind you," she'd told Mildred again and again. "Build yourself a new life, honey. Take up photography, or skiing . . . whatever. Get yourself a boyfriend—how about a handsome young lifeguard?"

"Don't be ridiculous," said Mildred.

But Ellie had kept after her. As a matter of fact, today's visit to the Archway Medical Center was the latest step in Ellie's continuing campaign to help her sister resuscitate her shattered life.

"Dr. Forrest did wonders for me, sheer wonders!" Ellie had told Mildred again and again during the past year. "Do what I did, sweetie. A quick chin tuck and maybe a little bit of breast augmentation . . . hey, I guarantee, you'll be astonished by the results!

"I feel ten years younger, Mildred, and you can, too. And the procedure takes less than an hour. They put you under a general anesthetic—it's completely painless. You wake up after about 45 minutes or so, and when you take that first look at yourself in his full-length mirror: wow!"

Fearful and cautious, Mildred had hung back at first. But Ellie had finally managed to win her over. And now, as the two of them sat beneath the dripping awning, the visitor from Minneapolis was beginning to feel a little of her sister's excitement.

"Tell you what," said Ellie, as she removed the keys from the ignition and tossed them into her leather handbag. "Once Dr. Forrest finishes with you and you've had a week or so to recover, we're going to Red Lobster and order the 'Shrimp Blowout.' My treat! You still love shrimp broiled with garlic, don't you?"

Mildred smiled in spite of herself. "I sure do."

"And that's not all," said Ellie. "I've already made you an appointment at The Razor's Edge. You're all set for tomorrow morning, 11 o'clock. If you lighten up that gorgeous blonde hair a little, and get it cut short and sexy . . . why, you'll be fighting the guys off with a stick!"

Mildred's smile broadened. "Don't be silly, dear. I'm 44 years old."

Ellie took her hand, squeezed it. "Listen, you're a spring chicken, sweetheart. Let's face it: you've still got those liquid green eyes, and you've still got that famous killer smile. Trust me: your new life as the Minnesota Bombshell is only getting *started*."

****

Dr. Larson Forrest was a tall, lean, thoughtful-looking man with flecks of silver scattered through his stylishly cut hair. He wore a charcoal-gray suit, top of the line at Armani, with a tiny white rosebud pinned to the lapel.

"Hi, Ellie. Great to see you again!"

"Hi, Dr. Forrest."

The plastic surgeon swung his blue-eyed gaze over to the newcomer. "You must be Mildred. Hello! Before I say anything else, I want you to know that your sister's been singing your praises to me for the past several weeks."

Mildred lit up, then tried to wave the compliment away. "Don't listen to her, Dr. Forrest—she's highly prejudiced!"

The beaming physician sent up a light-hearted chuckle. "Mildred, I enjoyed talking with you on the phone last week, and I hope I answered all your questions." Without waiting for her to respond, he rushed ahead, "If you'll follow me, I want you to meet the nurse anesthetist who'll be helping me during today's procedure. Do you remember me mentioning Nurse Karr on the phone?"

"I do," said Mildred.

Still smiling, the plastic surgeon led the way through a pair of gold-painted swinging doors and into the surgical suite, where a white-clad nurse was busily arranging a tray full of glittering instruments.

"Ellie, I'm sure you remember Sally Karr?"

"I certainly do," boomed Ellie, returning the nurse's cheerful wave. "It's great to see you again, Sally."

"Likewise," said Nurse Karr. "Goodness gracious, is it already two years since we did your procedure, Ellie?"

"That's right," grinned Ellie. "Time really flies, doesn't it?"

Now Dr. Forrest pointed the two visitors toward a pair of low-slung, avocado-colored chairs. "Ladies, if you'll settle back and relax, I'll take you quickly through the procedure we're going to follow. First of all, after we get Mildred nice and comfortable, Sally will hook her up to an IV and administrator the general anesthetic. It's a mild substance, very safe . . . and usually without side effects. Right, Ellie?"

"I never felt a thing," said Ellie.

"Millions of people receive it every year without any harm whatsoever."

He sent the patient his best smile. "Don't worry, Mildred, you won't be under the anesthetic for much more than 30 minutes—and Sally here is trained and licensed to take good care of you. She may even sing you a lullaby, as you drift off to dreamland!"

Everybody laughed.

"You're not nervous, are you?" asked Dr. Forrest.

"No, I'm not. Well . . . maybe a *little*."

Everybody laughed again.

"I'm not worried about the procedure," said Mildred. "Ellie has already explained that it's painless and safe. No, the only thing I'm worried about right now is how I'm gonna *look*, once I wake up!"

Gales of laughter all around. Smiling contentedly, Dr. Forrest was fingering the white rosebud in his lapel. He *liked* this new patient, and he certainly intended to do his best by her.

After a few more minutes of light-hearted banter, Ellie told her sister goodbye and headed off to the nearby Wal-Mart to buy some new screens for her back porch. "I'll see you guys in about an hour," she told them as she reached into her leather bag for her car keys. "I can't wait to see the results!"

Dr. Forrest nodded and smiled. "Don't worry about a thing," he told the departing Ellie. "We'll take good care of your sister . . . and when we finish with her, she's going to look like a million bucks!"

****

At first, everything went smoothly, and the cosmetic surgical procedure began to unfold like clockwork.

After making the patient comfortable on the surgical table and moving her equipment into position, Nurse Karr gently inserted a needle into her left arm near the elbow and then attached it to a line that ran from the IV bag hanging above her. Once the IV was started, the nurse anesthetist stood by to begin the first phase of general anesthesia, the "induction" phase, in which a number of different drugs (whether inhaled or pumped into the patient via an IV line) can be employed to bring the patient to a state of unconsciousness.

On this occasion, Nurse Karr would be using an anesthetic "cocktail"—a powerful combination of two hypnotic sedatives named propofol and ketamine—that could be counted on to put the patient into a deep sleep within about ten seconds. During more than 10 years of practice, Dr. Forrest had come to prefer these two agents for the initial sedation of the patient, since they greatly reduced the second, or "excitement" phase, during which some patients will experience muscle contractions, vomiting and sometimes even violent thrashing and irregular heartbeat.

Not to worry, however: Dr. Forrest had long ago discovered that most patients who were given the propofol and ketamine cocktail would glide peacefully through the excitement phase and quickly enter the third phase, known as the "surgical plane."

Once Mildred Harbison entered this phase, Dr. Forrest knew that it would be easy to keep her motionless and unconscious, by administering further small doses of propofol every 15 minutes or so, while monitoring her vital signs and changes in eye reflexes and pupil size in order to avoid overdose.

And so it began.

Leaning over the supine patient, Sally Karr gave her a brilliant smile. "Anytime you're ready, Mildred, I'll do my little thing and introduce you to the Sandman. Pleasant dreams, now!"

Mildred sent her a brave smile. "Ready when you are!"

Sally nodded, and squeezed the plunger on the hypodermic needle she held in her right hand. Transparent and invisible, the drug cocktail flowed swiftly into the IV line. A few seconds passed. Then Mildred asked: "Say, don't you want me to count out loud?"

The surgeon laughed. "Not necessary," said the genial Dr. Forrest. "But go right ahead, if you'd like. Bet you can't make it to six."

"Okay," said Mildred. "One, two, three . . ."—but her eyelids were fluttering now, and the word "four" came out as a whisper.

Then she was silent.

"Okay," said Dr. Forrest. He was no longer smiling. "I'm ready to start, as soon as you get her stabilized."

The patient lay motionless, with her eyelids still fluttering slightly.

She had no idea, as her general anesthesia began to take hold in earnest, that the "nurse anesthetist," the easygoing and laughter-loving 26-year-old Sally Karr, was a mere RN without any special training in anesthesia. She didn't know, either, that Dr. Forrest had actually met Nurse Karr for the first time only about two years before this moment, or that their original meeting place had been The Cat's Eye Pub, a popular watering hole for swinging singles, located just off the scenic highway that flanked Pensacola Bay.

Nurse Karr was actually Dr. Forrest's girlfriend, and she knew nothing more about administering general anesthesia than the little bit he had taught her so far.

Nor did the now-paralyzed and unconscious Mildred Harbison know that Dr. Forrest's earlier telephone promise to provide a "a qualified anesthesiologist" had been completely fraudulent.

Worst of all, she didn't know that the plastic surgeon—a frequent visitor to Las Vegas whose finances were in serious disarray—had fallen so far behind on his malpractice insurance premiums that his coverage had been terminated by his insurer, three weeks before Mildred Harbison arrived in his reception room at the Archway Medical Center.

Mildred knew none of these things, and now it was too late to consider them.

Her surgery was already underway.

****

Truth, Lies and the OR

Things went very well, at first. After easing Mildred through the induction and excitement phases of anesthesia and then establishing a trouble-free surgical plane, Nurse Karr settled back on her chair to watch the gifted surgeon do his stuff. Intent on showing off his skills to his good-looking girlfriend, the freewheeling Dr. Forrest employed his glittering scalpel with a flourish. Within a matter of five or six minutes, the key incisions for the breast implants had been made, and the augmentation procedure was well underway.

The mood in the doctor's surgical suite was light-hearted and jovial. While the stereo system played mellow Golden Oldies—bright, upbeat tunes like *I Got You, Babe* and *California Dreamin'*—the doctor and his RN girlfriend joked about a recent episode of *ER* they'd watched the night before, while enjoying several piña coladas on the balcony of the surgeon's Escambia Bay condo.

So relaxed and easygoing was their approach to the surgery, in fact, that Sally Karr even paused—once the patient's anesthesia had been stabilized—to stroll over to the portable refrigerator beside the window and grab two ice-cold bottles of Diet Cherry Pepsi. Sipping her soft drink and chatting with the skilled surgeon, she kept one eye on the patient's vital signs, while leaning against the operating table where the swift incisions were now taking place.

They were 22 minutes into the cosmetic procedure when the first sign of a potential problem emerged.

Deeply anesthetized now, the patient lay utterly still on the table . . . so still, in fact, that Dr. Forrest felt a slight flicker of concern. "Sally, can you give me a pulse rate, please?"

The nurse put her Pepsi can down and went to work. Within a minute or so, she was back with results. "She's slowing down, Win. *Way* down. I'm getting about 46, that's all."

The surgeon looked up from his work. "You're kidding."

"Nope, that was the count, all right. And she feels a little cold. Her skin feels a little clammy."

The doctor frowned. "Okay, no problem, we're almost there. Another seven, eight minutes should do it."

Sally stared at him. "Should I keep the drip going, then?"

The plastic surgeon thought for a moment. "Yeah . . . we're close to being finished. I don't think we're pushing the envelope. Keep the anesthesia going, same rate."

But five minutes later, he began to wonder if the envelope *had* been pushed. "She's down around 40, Win."

"Are you serious?" There were tiny beads of perspiration on his forehead now. "That's not supposed to be happening, Sally. Are you sure you've got it right?"

Sally nodded. "I am. I am. And she's pretty cold, Win."

He grimaced. "Eye reflex?"

A pause. Then: "I'm getting nothing."

By now the patient's respiration rate had also slowed, and her pupils had contracted to tiny pinpoints—often a warning that the individual is beginning to experience heart failure.

"I don't know, Win," said Sally. "This just doesn't *look* right. Do you . . . do you think we might need some help?"

He glared at her. "Help? What kind of help? What are you talking about?"

Sally lowered her eyes. "Well, I just meant . . . you know. You don't think she'll arrest, do you?"

****

Months later, the medical evidence would show clearly that the patient had, indeed, "arrested" on the operating table during her office-based surgery, and that the plastic surgeon, determined to finish his

Truth, Lies and the OR

botched procedure, had ordered the alarmed RN to continue the anesthesia for a few more minutes, regardless.

The Emergency Medical Technicians (EMTs) who were eventually called to the scene testified that the angry physician had demanded that he be allowed to "finish my damn operation" before the ambulance crew moved the obviously arrested patient to the ER at the nearest hospital, Pensacola General.

According to the medical record, in fact, the EMTs actually found it necessary to point out that they would summon local police in order to have the patient removed, if the enraged surgeon did not relent.

****

After loading the new porch screens from Wal-Mart into the back of her Toyota, Ellie cruised back to Myrtle Grove Road to pick up her sister and take her home for a good long rest.

But that trip home never took place.

Arriving at the Archway Clinic, Ellie was startled to see two Escambia County ambulances parked beside the facility. Their blue flashers were whirling, and, as she stepped from her car, Ellie could hear the radio blasting from one of the emergency vehicles, loud and clear:

> *Twenty-niner, this is Mobile Seven. We're moving the patient to Pensacola General, ASAP. Looks like she arrested during minor surgery at her doctor's office. We've got very little pulse, and BP is way down. Over.*
>
> *Copy that, Mobile Seven. Have you started IV adrenalin? Epinephrine? Over.*
>
> *Just hooked the line in a second ago. We're up and running with both, Control. Looks like she went into respiratory arrest during plastic surgery—and the doc fought us for a while. Said he wanted to complete the procedure. Bad news—we*

nearly had to bring in the Pensacola Police. But we're rolling now. Over.

Copy, Mobile Seven. We're Code Blue in ER, and standing by. Over and out.

Elie stood frozen on the sidewalk for a moment. "Oh my God . . . !"

Then she began to run.

But she'd taken only a few steps when the front doors of the clinic banged open. Stunned, Ellie watched two EMTs rolling a wheeled stretcher toward the nearest ambulance.

Mildred was on the stretcher.

Her eyes were closed, and her face was chalky-white.

Crazed with fear, Ellie staggered toward the two men in the blue denim uniforms with the red *EMT* patches.

"What happened? What happened? My God, that's my sister! Did something happen to her during surgery?"

The two men ignored her at first. They were busy moving the stretcher into the ambulance. "Mildred!" Ellie shouted, lurching in closer. "Mildred, can you hear me? I'm right here, honey; don't worry, I'm right here beside you!"

Was this a nightmare, or was it really happening? With her heart pounding violently, Ellie stepped up to the back door of the ambulance. "Can you tell me what happened? Did she . . . was there a problem? Is she bleeding? Will she be okay? Please *help* me!"

One of the attendants turned to her for a moment. "I'm sorry, ma'am, but we're not permitted to comment on medical issues." The technician gazed sadly at her. He was a pleasant-looking young man with mild blue eyes. "We gotta go," he said gently, "but you might want to speak with the doctor at the Archway Clinic. He knows what happened.

"It's a Dr. Forrest. Winston Forrest. Do you know him?"

"My God," she moaned. "I do."

The EMT slammed the back door shut, then ran toward the front of the ambulance, which was already moving.

Ellie stood alone in the street now.

It had begun to rain again, but she didn't notice. The wind rose and there was a rumble of distant thunder. Should she run upstairs and confront the doctor, or should she hurry to the hospital—Pensacola General—to look after her poor sister as best she could?

The answer was obvious.

Sobbing and nearly hysterical, she climbed back into the Toyota and began the heart-breaking ride to the hospital ER, where a dozen intensive-care specialists were about to begin fighting for Mildred Harbison's life.

Their heroic efforts lasted for several days.

But the patient had suffered major brain damage during the lengthy period in which her respiration had broken down. Comatose and utterly unresponsive, she hovered for a few days in a twilight condition at the boundary line between life and death.

Ellie was sitting beside her sister, one week after the botched "chin tuck and breast augmentation," when she breathed her last.

****

Almost exactly seven months after the death of his patient due to "respiratory arrest and subsequent severe brain injury" (the medical account of death provided by the Escambia County Coroner), Dr. Winston Forrest went into Chapter 11 bankruptcy proceedings.

The legal procedure was a sham, however; its real purpose had been to protect the physician from any lawsuit damages that might arise from a malpractice action in the accidental death of Mildred Harbison of Minneapolis, Minnesota, during her disastrous office-based surgery.

After analyzing the prospects for recovering significant monetary damages from a physician who was now bankrupt and penniless, Ellie's Pensacola attorney advised against legal action. In the end, she decided not to file the $20 million malpractice lawsuit that she had hoped would provide compensation to Mildred's devastated son and daughter. In a final, bitter irony, she felt obligated to pay the legal costs which had already been incurred—more than $5,000—out of her own pocket.

Of course, Dr. Winston Forrest had long departed the State of Florida by then and may now be practicing plastic surgery in another state, since the laws that currently regulate the practice of office-based surgery do not require surgeons or anesthesia providers to supply licensing authorities with reports of accidental patient deaths or injuries that have occurred during prior operations.

Ellie accompanied her sister's body back to Minnesota for burial, and did her best to comfort Mildred's two children.

To this day, whenever it rains in Pensacola and the sky turns dark with another rumbling thunderstorm from the nearby Gulf of Mexico, Ellie thinks of her sister.

If only we'd known, she tells herself. *If only we'd been warned about the risks we were taking that day.*

Rx: Be a careful, informed consumer before undergoing any office-based surgery

As of this writing (Jan. 2008) approximately 25% of all surgery in this country is done in an office setting. And, according to experts, it will continue to rise in numbers. We are not just talking about the cosmetic, plastic, and dental surgery that has been done in offices for over 30 years. Already, surgical procedures including inguinal hernia repairs, hemorrhoidectomies, liposuction, and breast augmentations are being done in office settings. In the near future, this list is expected to broaden to include abdominal and vaginal hysterectomies, laparoscopic gallbladders, diagnostic laparoscopic surgery, mastectomies, lumbar and cervical diskectomies, anterior cruciate ligament repairs, and ENT procedures, to name a few.

What makes office-based surgery potentially such a high risk is that, as of this writing, only 22 states have any type of standards or guidelines in place to attempt to ensure that the quality of care and safety in office-based surgery will be equal to that in an ambulatory surgery center or hospital. These states include Alabama, California, Colorado, Connecticut, Florida, Illinois, Kansas, Louisiana, Massachusetts, Mississippi, New Jersey, New York, North Carolina, Ohio, Oklahoma, Oregon, Pennsylvania, Rhode Island, South Carolina, Tennessee, Texas, and Virginia. In all other states, once the office door is closed, what goes on behind closed doors is the sole business of that surgeon. Consequently, there are NO ongoing quality control or peer review processes taking place in that office similar to what is required in every hospital and ambulatory surgery center in this country. Without these two processes, the state and national accreditations that are required for these medical facilities to operate would be withheld.

To put the relative risks of office-based surgery into perspective, we need only to go to a study completed in 2002 by Dr. Hector Vila from the University of South Florida in Tampa. He compared the number of complications and deaths from surgeries done in office-based surgery versus ambulatory surgery centers for a two-year period (2000–2002) in Florida. He found there was a tenfold increase in both complications and deaths for surgeries done in office-based settings over ambulatory surgery centers. Had this study been a comparison between office-based surgery and hospital surgery, the disparity would have been even greater. Furthermore, Florida is a state that has strong guidelines to ensure safety and quality of care in the office surgical setting and these had already been in place for several years prior to the time of this study. Yet, in spite of the guidelines, these alarming results were found.

Regardless of these crucial facts, the insurance companies are jumping on the band wagon to promote office-based surgery. Why? It is simple economics. These facilities charge fees that are lower than in any other setting. Who else benefits from office-based surgery? When surgery is performed in a hospital or ambulatory surgery center, the surgeon only receives his/her professional fee for performing the surgery. However, in office-based surgery, the surgeon also receives a profit on the facility fee. Furthermore, if an anesthesiologist is not involved with the IV (intravenous) sedation/anesthesia being given, the surgeon may also be making a profit in that area. Recently, at the American Society of Anesthesiologists' Annual Meeting, a plastic surgeon form the Harvard Staff admitted publicly, "Make no bones about it, surgeons are double-dipping when doing office-based surgery." One can easily take this a step further and say that triple-dipping is often going on when the profit from IV sedation/anesthesia is factored in. It is quite evident why surgeons are also pushing this type care—more profit and fewer restrictions on what they can do.

Where are patients' rights in all of this? Obviously, this is another area where the insurance companies are allowing safe patient care to take a back seat to decreased costs and higher profits. Furthermore, it is an area where physicians' motives for medical decisions can be open to question. Bottom line profits may take priority over top quality care.

As of this writing, a patient still has the right to refuse an office setting for most surgical procedures, and instead, opt for a hospital or ambulatory surgery center. The surgical procedure may be appropriate for an office setting, but the patient's medical condition may make the patient an inappropriate candidate for surgery in an office setting. Such conditions as major coronary artery disease with unstable or significant angina, major diabetes, significant pulmonary disease, major hypertension, obesity, and sleep apnea may all easily make the office surgical setting inappropriate. In fact, the hospital outpatient surgery department may provide the safest setting for your surgery. Should you get into trouble, you don't have to go through a transfer to a hospital and all the ancillary services are immediately available for your care. Do your homework, make wise choices, and do not be talked into a surgical setting that you instinctively feel is wrong for you.

As Dr. Vila's article indicates, there are a number of reasons why office-based surgery may be dangerous. Certainly at the top of the list is the type of IV sedation/anesthesia utilized and the qualifications of the people who administer this. Reports keep surfacing across the country that non-medical personnel, such as office managers and secretaries, are administering IV medications for sedation. The monitoring of the patient's vital signs is then being done by the same person who is doing the surgery, dental work, or diagnostic procedure. This is indeed "pushing the envelope" to the limits.

The practice of employing IV sedation for surgery, especially for surgery done under local anesthesia, is very common in today's practice of medicine. The primary purpose of this sedation is to allow patients to tolerate surgery or unpleasant procedures by relieving anxiety, discomfort, and/or pain in a safe manner. This type sedation has found its niche particularly in outpatient surgery especially in ambulatory surgery centers and office-based surgical settings. **Make no mistake about it: IV sedation is a form of anesthesia and must be administered and monitored accordingly**. Unfortunately, more than a few physicians and dentists play down this important point when discussing with patients their upcoming surgery and type of sedation to be given.

There are two distinct types of IV sedation: conscious and unconscious. In conscious sedation, the patient is able to easily respond to verbal command and does not lose his/her reflexes, especially the important ability to swallow. With deep or unconscious sedation, the patient does not respond to verbal command and does not retain the all important swallowing reflex. This is the reflex that helps to prevent aspirating any stomach contents that may come up. And aspiration pneumonia still carries a very high mortality rate of 90% or greater. **It is extremely important to understand there can be a very fine line between conscious sedation and unconscious sedation.** Furthermore, very often what starts out as conscious sedation ends up as unconscious sedation either inadvertently or deliberately. In many cases this is done knowingly and deliberately. Herein lie the potential dangers.

In addition to this, much of today's IV sedation utilizes the drug propofol (Diprovan). From an anesthesiologist's perspective, there is no such thing as conscious sedation with propofol. It is unconscious sedation! Additionally, the use of a sedative drug such as Versed or Valium and/or a narcotic such as Demerol, morphine, or fentanyl in combination with propofol, further ensures an unconscious sedation. Finally, at the present time, we do not have a reversal drug for propofol.

Much of today's conscious sedation is being done in areas outside of the operating room. Besides office-based settings, another area where much IV sedation is employed is in diagnostic laboratories such as the GI labs (gastrointestinal). In many of these settings, conscious sedation is being administered by personnel other than those fully trained and certified in anesthesia. This means RNs/LPNs, and/or nurses' aides may be giving this sedation and monitoring the patient. In many cases, the physician or dentist doing the procedure is administering the sedation and monitoring the patient at the same time. This can be a potentially dangerous situation especially when conscious sedation becomes unconscious/deep sedation.

As of this writing, many of the 22 states with guidelines in place for office-based surgery do address unconscious/deep sedation and who must administer it. The standard requires that a person fully trained and currently certified in anesthesia must give this type sedation and monitor the patient. Simply stated, a certified registered nurse anesthetist or an anesthesiologist must be that person. However, there is no such stipulation regarding who can administer conscious sedation.

Unfortunately, many physicians and dentists get around the sedation regulation by telling patients they will have conscious sedation for their procedure. If you have had a procedure under "conscious sedation" and do not remember a single thing afterwards, the chances are great your sedation was unconscious, and you may not have had the proper medical personnel involved. Many gastroscopes, and office-based plastic surgeries are done under sedation without an anesthesia personnel present. **Make no mistake: the physician or dentist is making a profit from that sedation when no anesthesia personnel are involved.**

You as the patient must ask questions ahead of time about the sedation you will be receiving, and who will administer it and monitor you. If anesthesia personnel are not going to be involved or are not in the facility where your procedure/surgery is being done, your medical interests and safety might better be served by changing to a facility where anesthesia personnel are present.

The initial recovery from IV sedation, especially unconscious sedation, is another critical period where patient observation and monitoring of the vital signs are essential. These are best accomplished by nursing personnel who are trained in critical care, including management of the airway of a sedated or comatose patient. Many office-based surgical practices lack this type of skilled personnel. Ask questions, get complete answers, and be sure this office setting is patient-friendly for office-based surgery.

In the past decade or so, we have seen an explosion in this country of increasing numbers of "medical spas." These medical spas are combining manicures, massage therapy, and facials—which historically have been offered by a day spa—with Botox injections, laser treatments, and other more complicated procedures which normally require medical supervision. Some of these spas are free-standing, with physicians on staff, while others have no physicians present on the premises. It's an ambiguous situation: is it a spa or a doctor's office? Since these medical spas may not be designated as true doctors' offices, they do not come under any state guidelines/regulations, or only under minimal ones at best. Medical spas are big business! In 2006 gross volume of business was projected to be over $1 billion. The baby boomers are largely fueling the demand for this type of service.

Certainly two key issues clouding this industry are: what does it mean to provide "medical supervision," and how much can one person legitimately supervise? Does one supervise by being on the premises, supervise from another geographic location, or supervise over the telephone? These are all key questions that you the consumer should ask and for which you should have answers before EVER signing a consent for treatment. Once you have gathered your information, you will need to decide if the risks are worth taking or whether your medical safety would be better served in a different type setting.

Remember: knowledge is your best defense to help prevent a medical disaster. As a patient, know your rights, and do not compromise them!

IN SUMMARY

- Approximately 25% of all U.S. surgeries are performed in an office setting. Not only is the share of surgeries in office settings expected to increase in the future, but the types of surgeries performed in office settings are projected to significantly broaden.

- Only 22 states (as of this writing) have any type of standards or guidelines attempting to ensure that the quality of care and safety in office-based surgery will be equal to that in an ambulatory surgery center or hospital.

- A patient has the right to refuse an office setting for most surgical procedures and elect to have surgery in a hospital or ambulatory surgery center.

- A patient's medical condition may make the patient an inappropriate candidate for surgery in the office setting even though the surgical procedure might otherwise be appropriate. Such conditions include major coronary artery disease with unstable or significant angina, major diabetes, significant pulmonary disease, major hypertension, obesity, and sleep apnea.

- The relative risk of office-based surgery is impacted by the type of IV sedation/anesthesia utilized and the qualifications of the people who administer it.

- You need to ask questions prior to surgery about the sedation you will be receiving and the qualifications of who will administer it and monitor you. If anesthesia personnel are not going to be involved or are not in the facility where your procedure/surgery is being done, your medical interests and safety might better be served by changing to a facility where anesthesia personnel are present.

F. W. Ernst, M.D. — William G. Pace III, M. D.

OFFICE-BASED SURGERY QUESTIONS

Here are 11 very important questions for which you should have complete answers before signing a consent for surgery in a physician's office. If you can not get complete answers or you are leery of any answer, then that physician's office may well not be "patient friendly" for office-based surgery and IV sedation/anesthesia.

1. Does the surgeon have privileges to do the same procedure in a nearby hospital or outpatient surgery center? (within 5-10 miles) If not, WHY?
2. Has the surgeon's privileges to do this same procedure ever been denied, withdrawn, or put on probation at any medical facility? If so, WHY?
3. Who will sedate me or give me anesthesia? Is this person fully trained and certified by the appropriate anesthesia organization? (American Association for Nurse Anesthetists for C.R.N.A.; American Board of Anesthesiologists for M.D. or D.O.) Furthermore, when will I have my pre-op visit with these anesthesia personnel? (Hopefully, this visit is done at least 24 hours prior to surgery.)
4. Will the individual administering my IV sedation and/or anesthesia be in constant attendance with me during the surgery? A MUST!
5. Is the anesthesia machine a current model and similar to the machines used in nearby hospitals and ambulatory surgery centers? Is the machine serviced properly and in a timely manner? (quarterly a year)
6. Will the monitors used on me during my anesthetic and in the recovery room be the same as would be used if I were having

my operation in a hospital or ambulatory surgery center? If not, WHY!

7. Who will recover me following surgery in the recovery area? Is this person an RN trained and with experience in critical care nursing, including management of the airway of a sedated or comatose patient? If not, WHY!

8. Is the physician's office fully equipped to handle any type of medical emergency? Is this equipment checked weekly and kept up to date? Are the personnel trained to handle these emergencies including at least one physician on the premise at all times who is ACLS certified? If the answer is no to any part of this question, WHY?

9. How are the surgical instruments sterilized after each surgery and do all personnel having patient contact wear appropriate surgical attire?

10. Are arrangements in place for immediate transfer and admission to a nearby hospital (within 10 miles) if any unexpected complications arise or if I am unable to go home following my surgery for any reason? A MUST!

11. Is this surgeon's office accredited by one of the three main medical accrediting organizations in this country? These are JCAHO (Joint Commission for Accreditation of HealthCare Organizations), AAAHC (Accreditation Association for Ambulatory HealthCare), and AAAASF (American Association for Accreditation of Ambulatory Surgery Facilities). If not, BEWARE!

F. W. Ernst, M.D. — William G. Pace III, M. D.

"10 Core Principles for Office-based Surgery"
Formulated and Unanimously Passed by the American Medical Association, November 2003

In March, 2003, a Committee on Office-based Surgery, made up of members from the American Medical Association (AMA) and the American College of Surgeons (ACS), drafted and unanimously passed 10 Core Principles to regulate office-based surgery in this country. These Principles are meant to ensure that the quality of surgical care in an office setting will equal that in an ambulatory surgery center (one day surgery center) or a hospital. The AMA House of Delegates at its 2003 annual Meeting referred these Core Principles to its Board of Trustees (BOT) for a decision. In late November, 2003, the BOT unanimously approved these Principles for office-based surgery essentially unchanged. This means these Principles will help formulate what the standard of care will become in this country for office-based surgery.

At the present time, only 22 states have standards in place to regulate office-based surgery. Unfortunately, the standards in some of these 22 states do not measure up to or equal these Core Principles the AMA has passed. Before you seek surgical treatment in an office setting, you should become familiar with these Principles. Find out if your state has standards in place for office-based surgery and how do these standards measure up to the Core Principles passed by the AMA. **This is especially important if your surgery will require any kind of intravenous sedation, general anesthesia, or major block anesthesia.**

Presently, **NO** medical insurance plan can require you to have your surgery in an office setting. Know your rights and be fully knowledgeable before you ever sign a consent for office-based surgery and anesthesia. Below are the 10 Core Principles as passed by the AMA. The term moderate sedation equals "conscious intravenous sedation" and deep sedation equals "unconscious intravenous sedation."

Core Principle #1: Guidelines or regulations for office-based surgery should be developed by states according to levels of anesthesia defined by the American Society of Anesthesiologists (ASA) excluding local anesthesia or minimal sedation.

Core Principle #2: Physicians should select patients for office-based surgery using moderate sedation/deep sedation, or general anesthesia by criteria including the ASA Physical Status Classification System and so document.

Core Principle #3: Physicians who perform office-based surgery using moderate sedation, deep sedation, or general anesthesia should have their facilities accredited by the Joint Commission on Accreditation of HealthCare Organizations (JCAHO), Accreditation Association for Ambulatory Health Care (AAAHC), American Association for Accreditation of Ambulatory Surgical Facilities (AAAASF), American Osteopathic Association (AOA), or by a state recognized entity, such as the Institute for Medical Quality (IMQ), or be state licensed and/or Medicare certified.

Core Principle #4: Physicians performing office-based surgery with moderate sedation, deep sedation, or general anesthesia must have admitting privileges at a nearby hospital, or a transfer agreement with another physician who has admitting privileges at a nearby hospital, or maintain an emergency transfer agreement with a nearby hospital.

Core Principle #5: States should follow the guidelines outlined by the Federation of State Medical Boards (FSMB) regarding informed consent.

Core Principle #6: For office surgery with moderate sedation, deep sedation, or general anesthesia, states should consider legally privileged adverse incident reporting requirements as recommended by the FSMB and accompanied by periodic peer review and a program of Continuous Quality Improvement.

Core Principle #7: Physicians performing office-based surgery using moderate sedation, deep sedation, or general anesthesia must obtain and maintain Board Certification by one of the Boards recognized by the American Board of Medical Specialties, American Osteopathic Association, or a board with equivalent standards approved by the state medical board within 5 years of completing an approved residency training program. The procedure must be one that is generally recognized by that certifying board as falling within the scope of training and practice of the physician providing the care.

Core Principle #8: Physicians performing office-based surgery with moderate sedation, deep sedation, or general anesthesia may show competency by maintaining core privileges at an accredited or licensed hospital or ambulatory surgical center, for the procedures they perform in the office setting. Alternatively, the governing body of the office facility is responsible for a peer review process for privileging physicians based on nationally recognized credentialing standards.

Core Principle #9: For office-based surgery with moderate sedation, deep sedation, or general anesthesia, at least one physician who is credentialed or currently recognized as having successfully completed a course in advanced resuscitative techniques (e.g. ATLS, ACLS, or PALS), must be present or immediately available with age-and-size appropriate resuscitative equipment until the patient has met the criteria for discharge from the facility. In addition, other medical personnel with direct patient contact should at a minimum be trained in Basic Cardiac Life Support (BCLS).

Core Principle #10: Physicians administering or supervising moderate sedation, deep sedation, or general anesthesia should have appropriate education and training.

F. W. Ernst, M.D. — William G. Pace III, M. D.

CHAPTER NINE

AWARENESS UNDER GENERAL ANESTHESIA

Dr. Ernst

KEY POINT:

- In 2005 and 2006, an estimated twenty- to forty-thousand U.S. patients experienced some degree of awareness under general anesthesia each year. This "awareness" can include feeling pain related to surgery while they are under general anesthesia.

A Nightmare in Tunica

The patient was undergoing surgery to repair a fractured ankle, and his surgeon was halfway through a grueling procedure that called for attaching a supportive plate to the broken bone with metal screws. But what the surgeon didn't know was that the man on the table had suddenly awakened from his general anesthesia. Paralyzed by the intravenous drugs that had been pumped into his system, however, the patient was unable to move a single muscle.

With growing horror, the man beneath the scalpel realized that he could feel the first metal screw beginning to turn against his inflamed and keenly sensitive ankle. A moment later, as he lay helpless and desperate, the nightmare began.

A man and his loyal dog! Is there any joy like it?

They were hiking together, on that mild afternoon in May, along a hillside trail surrounded by sunlit willow oaks and breezy red maples.

Now Jack Perkins held up the knobby stick he'd just retrieved from beneath the scarlet blossoms of a flowering trumpet honeysuckle. Tantalizingly, he waggled the stick beneath the nose of the panting black Labrador.

"Okay, Shadow, are you ready to *run*?"

The dog crouched expectantly at his master's feet. The mellow sunshine gleamed in his honey-brown eyes.

"Go!"

Airborne, the knobby stick hurtled through the air, with Shadow in hot pursuit.

It was 3:30 on a Saturday afternoon in 2005, and Jack Perkins was already sold on the joys of retirement. After spending the past 20 years as the President and CEO at Southland Communications, an international information-technology company based in his native Tunica, Mississippi, the hard-charging Perkins had turned 65 only a few months before. At his wife's urging—and after a great deal of internal debate—he had finally decided to turn the reins of the giant computer company over to a younger executive.

Now, having settled into a graceful Victorian-style country house located about 20 miles south of Tunica, he was taking a few months to catch his breath and review his prospects before deciding on the best way to enjoy his hard-earned retirement.

Accompanied by the endlessly energetic Shadow, Perkins loved to wander along the hilly trails and walking paths that honeycombed the forestlands near his home. Day after day, he and the black Lab drifted among the budding swamp maples and the white-blossomed elderberry bushes that formed the botanical signature of this region of northwestern Mississippi.

Truth, Lies and the OR

While the squirrels cavorted merrily on the branches above their heads, Jack always kept an eye out for the majestic red-tailed hawk and counted himself especially lucky whenever he managed to spot one.

"Good dog!" he said now, as he took the knobby stick from the salivating jaws of his canine buddy. Walking side by side, the two of them were now making their way up a steep incline. A few feet to the left of the trail, a narrow creek babbled cheerfully, dappled here and there with mellow sunshine. "All right, Shadow," sang the jubilant retiree, leaning far back in order to get off a more powerful throw, "this time you're *really* going to run!"

But then it happened.

The leaves beneath the senior citizen's right foot had been soaked by the splashing brook, and they were slick as ice.

Perkins went down hard, and when he landed, his left ankle crashed against a large, anvil-shaped rock that flanked the trail at a steep angle.

Nothing moved for a few seconds. The dog was still crouched, still waiting for the throw. The spring breeze riffled through a patch of dark-green alligator weed beside the trail, as Jack struggled to push himself back up to his feet. He could hear a blue jay screaming in the distance: *Awk! Awk! Awk!*

He was standing upright again—but as soon as tried to take a step, he collapsed.

A single glance at his left ankle told him all he needed to know: He'd sprained it. Maybe even broken it. Each time he tried to move his left foot, waves of burning pain exploded from the ankle joint and raced all the way up to his knee. The foot had also gone completely numb, so that he was unable to turn it in any direction, or even to wiggle his toes.

What now? He was nearly two miles from his home on Green Branch Road. For a moment, he felt a wave of irrational panic: how was he going to get help, if he couldn't even move? But then his eyes lit up.

Thank heavens for Marge! Although he'd often accused her of acting like a "Nervous Nellie" and a "worry wart," Jack's wife had been absolutely insistent. Again and again she had nagged him, "Jack, I don't want you walking those trails without your cell phone. What if something goes wrong out there? What if you were to have an accident, or suddenly get sick?"

Because of the thoughtful Marge, Jack Perkins suddenly had an ace in his hand. Digging deep into the left pocket of his blue jeans, he quickly retrieved the silver-painted Alltel and dialed the number for his home.

Marge answered on the second ring.

"You *fell*, Jack? On the trail? Are you hurt?"

"No big deal," he said. "Just an annoyance, really—but my left ankle hit a rock and now it doesn't seem to work very well."

"All right," she said. "Just stay calm. I'm going to call 911 right now."

He chuckled. "Isn't that a bit melodramatic, Marge? Why not just ask Bill Rutledge to bring his all-terrain motorbike out here and pick me up?"

"No way," said Marge. He could imagine her frowning, shaking her head on the other end of the line. "I think the Rutledges are out of town, Jack. Besides, he's not a medical doctor. You don't want to aggravate that injury. No, this is a job for the professionals. Where are you, exactly?"

"I'm about two-thirds of the way up the hill above the Stone Chapel, right beside the creek. Right here on the main trail."

He looked up at the loyal Shadow, standing only a few feet away. The dog had begun to bark his head off.

"I'll be fine," he told Marge with a chuckle. "The EMTs will probably hear Shadow before they see us—he's gone into full guard-dog mode!"

Truth, Lies and the OR

"Fine," said Marge. "Now you stay still. Don't try to move, you hear me?"

"Ten-four, commander."

"Just sit tight, Jack. Help is on the way!"

They gave him the bad news in the Emergency Room. He'd broken the ankle in two places. "We can fly you up to Memphis to see a specialist," Dr. Harbell told him, "but I'm not sure that's really necessary.

"Do you know Bill Schultz? He's our main orthopedics guy—handles these kinds of injuries every day of the week. It looks to me like you're gonna need a plate and screws on that, and Bill has done that procedure hundreds of times over the years.

"It's your call, Jack, but I recommend that you get the procedure done right here at Tunica General."

Twenty-four hours later, they were wheeling him into the hospital's Number Three Surgical Suite, where two smiling nurses greeted him cheerfully.

A moment later, the swinging doors on the other side of the suite banged open, and a tall, broad-shouldered man in green surgical scrubs came gliding toward them.

"Jack, we're all set," boomed Dr. Schultz. "The anesthesiologist, Dr. Corso, will be along in a minute. I should point out that Dr. Corso is filling in for our regular anesthesia guy, Dr. Blair, who's down in Florida attending his daughter's college graduation."

"I understand," said Jack.

"Not to worry," said Dr. Schultz. He gave the patient an encouraging smile. "Dr. Corso happened to be in town for a medical conference, and we're lucky to get him. He comes highly recommended.

He happens to be the resident anesthesiologist at a regional VA Hospital over in Tennessee, so you can be sure he knows his stuff."

"No problem," said Jack.

Dr. Anthony Corso turned out to be a short, heavy set man with bushy eyebrows and pudgy hands. His cheeks were florid and there were deep, shadowy bags under his eyes. But he seemed at ease in the surgical suite, and quite friendly. After shaking hands with Jack Perkins, he explained that he would be supervising his general anesthesia during the ninety-minute operation. "We're going to use a very mild anesthetic—propofol, mostly—that's known to have very few side effects," said Dr. Corso. "You'll be in deep sleep after fifteen or twenty seconds, and it will be my job to keep you that way until the last stitches are in and you're ready for the recovery room.

"Don't worry, you won't feel a thing!"

Jack nodded, took a deep breath. "Okay, guys, let's go for it!"

What neither Jack Perkins nor Dr. Schultz knew, as the ankle-repair operation got underway, was that Dr. Anthony Corso had been struggling hard in his anesthesiology practice during the past several years.

After a painful divorce and a series of difficult financial setbacks triggered by an auto accident (two people had been seriously injured) in which he'd been cited for drunk-driving, Dr. Corso had found himself besieged by hungry lawyers who demanded sky-high fees. In order to pay them all off, he'd been loading up his schedule to the breaking point. In addition to running his own private practice, he'd recently stepped in as resident anesthesiologist at the VA hospital. And he was also taking on plenty of jobs like this one—a one-day assignment in a city where he happened to be visiting—in order to pay his mounting legal fees.

After more than two years of working 16-hour days, the 58-year-old Dr. Corso was approaching the point of exhaustion. And now, as he settled in beside Jack Perkins and prepared to begin moving the propofol into his bloodstream via the IV, the visiting physician could feel the fatigue tugging at his eyelids. Oh, well. In another 90 minutes or so, the ankle-repair would be completed and he could wash up and head for the airport.

"Are you comfortable, Jack?" Both doctors were now poised above him, looking relaxed and cheerful. "Ready to say good-night for a while?"

He nodded. And within 30 seconds, he was completely unconsciousness.

Dr. Corso nodded at his colleague. "Okay, we're in good shape, Bill. He's into the induction phase, no problem. You can gear up, and I'll give you the green light. Shouldn't be more than seven or eight minutes."

"Sounds good, Tony." Already gloved, the surgeon was contemplating the tray of glittering instruments before him. The two nurses had moved in closer, as well. During the next hour and a half, the four of them would work smoothly together. While the scalpel flashed and the metal screws bit deeply into the patient's bones, Jack Perkins would remain supine on the table, breathing gently and utterly motionless.

Displaying a steady heartbeat and healthy vital signs, the patient appeared to doing very well. In medical parlance, he was "sailing through the operation." But appearances (including even those provided by medical instruments) can sometimes be misleading—and in this case, they certainly were.

Forty-seven minutes into the surgical procedure, Jack Perkins began to wake up.

Had Dr. Corso underestimated the amount of anesthetic that would be required to keep the patient unconscious throughout the operation? Or had he nodded off mentally during the tedious 80 minutes while his patient lay dead to the world, and failed to provide each IV dose of anesthetic on its proper schedule?

To this day, no one can be sure.

What Jack Perkins *does* know for sure, however, is that he came to awareness somewhere in the middle of his operation.

For a few flashing seconds, he heard a buzzing in his ears. Then it subsided, to be followed by a man's voice: "Screws, please. Hey, I don't think we're going to need the drill, folks. Looks like the fracturel plane is already lined up for us."

A moment later, Perkins felt a stinging pain moving up his left leg, from the ankle toward the kneecap. *Damn . . . that hurts!*

But when he tried to open his eyes—tried to open his mouth—nothing happened.

Suddenly, he felt an icy gust of fear go surging through his brain. He was paralyzed. The wires were down. He couldn't move and he couldn't speak. And the doctors didn't know that.

What followed were 30 minutes of unspeakable hell! Again and again, Jack Perkins experienced the brutal, lacerating pain that accompanied the twisting of the metal screws into his naked bones.

Again and again, he tried to move a hand, a foot, even a finger. Nothing.

With each jab of the needle, as the sutures were slowly closed, he wanted to roar with the agony caused by the tearing and cutting of his helpless flesh.

But he couldn't speak. Or move. And it was another torturous seventeen minutes before the last stitches and bandages were in place and the suffering Jack Perkins was finally wheeled down the hallway to the Tunica General Hospital Recovery Room.

Two months later, the still-enraged retiree sat in his lawyer's office on Gloster Street in Tunica.

"Jack, I know you won't like this, but I'm gonna tell it like it is," said Avery Kanigel. "You don't have a case. Period. You don't have zilch. I'd love to take them on—you know that—but I'd be wasting your hard-earned money."

Perkins stared at him. "Avery, I can't believe it. Are you telling me there's nothing I can do?"

The lawyer shook his graying head. Sighed. "Look, we both know it was malpractice. Okay? I don't have the slightest doubt that you were awake throughout half of that operation, and that you suffered terribly as a result. But the standard for evidence for medical malpractice is pretty high in Mississippi, and we don't have much. It's your word against theirs, Jack, and they've got two docs and two nurses who will all say you don't know what the hell you're talking about."

Jack nodded glumly. "They already *did* say that, Avery. As soon as I began to complain, they told me that all I was *really* remembering were the first few minutes in the recovery room. They said it happens frequently—patients wake up, and they remember some pain, and they assume that the pain happened during the surgical procedure, when it actually took place only two or three minutes before that, right in recovery."

The lawyer was shaking his head in frustration. "You're making my point for me, Jack. To win in court, we'd have to convince a jury that your memory of that procedure was impeccable. But they'd claim otherwise, and they'd hit you with a ton of medical evidence."

He gave his client a long, mournful glance. "It's a non-starter, Jack. We can't win with it, okay? I know you're not a hunter, but we have a saying in Mississippi: That dog won't hunt!"

Jack Perkins began climbing to his feet.

"Okay. Thanks, Avery. I know you gave it your best."

To this day, whenever it rains in northwestern Mississippi, Jack Perkins feels the pain in his left ankle.

It's a dull, persistent, throbbing ache . . . and it always reminds him of the agony he experienced that day on the operating table at Tupelo General Hospital.

Every once in a while, when the rain is falling against the windows and his ankle misery flares, Jack will tell his loyal spouse about the anger and the frustration he still feels today.

"I wish I'd known in advance that anesthesia isn't an exact science," he will tell the sympathetic Marge. "If only I'd known that, I could have taken the proper precautions!"

Rx: Be aware of the factors and conditions that can increase your risk of intraoperative awareness

Over the past fifteen to twenty years, an increasing number of cases of awareness under general anesthesia has been reported. Awareness under general anesthesia is a situation where surgical patients can recall their surroundings, conversations in the OR, or even pain related to their surgery while they are under general anesthesia. Frighteningly, the incidence of intraoperative awareness is generally reported in 1-2 cases per 1000 general anesthetics. In 2005 and 2006, approximately twenty million general anesthetics were administered in this country each year. This would mean 20,000-40,000 patients experienced some degree of awareness under general anesthesia each year. When other types of anesthetics are used, such as local or regional anesthesia with or without intravenous sedation, it is expected and accepted that patients may experience awareness during the surgical procedure. However, if the local or block anesthesia is working correctly, the patient should not feel pain.

What are the potential patient risk factors for experiencing awareness under general anesthesia?

1. Any previous episode(s) of awareness
2. Patient substance use or abuse
3. Chronic-pain patients being treated with high doses of opioids
4. A history of or anticipated difficulty in placing the breathing tube
5. Medical conditions which place a patient at an increased risk for general anesthesia
6. Limited circulatory reserve (a decreased blood volume)

Surgical procedures that carry an increased risk for awareness under general anesthesia:

1. Cardiac surgery
2. Cesarean section
3. Trauma surgery
4. Emergency surgery

Type of anesthetic technique used that carries an increased incidence of awareness under general anesthesia:

1. Planned use of muscle relaxants during the maintenance phase of anesthesia
2. Total IV (intravenous) anesthesia
3. A nitrous oxide/opioid anesthetic
4. Reduction of anesthetic doses during the time of muscle paralysis

It is notable that the presence of some of these risk factors has been reported to increase the relative risk of awareness under general anesthesia to nearly 1% of patients.

F. W. Ernst, M.D. — William G. Pace III, M. D.

What can a surgical patient do to try to protect himself/herself against experiencing awareness under general anesthesia?

- First, be aware of the factors and conditions that can increase your risk of intraoperative awareness as listed above.
- Second, and very importantly, in your preoperative anesthesia visit, discuss with the anesthesia personnel your concerns about awareness under anesthesia and receive complete answers to your questions. Be sure you share with the anesthesia personnel any problems you have had with previous anesthetics, including past awareness.
- Third, be sure you make the anesthesia personnel aware of any prescription drugs or over-the-counter medications you are taking, and how long you have been taking any of these medicines.

It is important to point out that a preoperative anesthesia visit/consultation is included as part of the anesthesia fee charged for your anesthetic. With few exceptions, omission of an anesthesia preoperative evaluation is a breach of the standard of care.

During your preoperative anesthesia visit, you might wish to discuss the use of the new brain-activity monitor. If you are at an increased risk for awareness under general anesthesia, then you might wish to request the use of this monitor for your surgery. It is important to understand there are at least eight different brain activity monitors available on the market for use by anesthesia personnel. It is also important to understand that all these monitors are NOT the same.

At the present time, the BIS (Bi-spectral index) monitor has the extensive clinical studies/trials done to document and validate the results the developer claims. These studies conclude that when the BIS monitor is used during anesthesia, there is an 80% reduction in the occurrence of awareness under general anesthesia. When you are discussing anesthesia awareness in your pre-operative visit, it might be helpful to inquire which brain activity monitor is used at the medical facility at which your surgery will be performed. If it is not the BIS monitor, then you will have to decide whether or not you are comfortable with some other type brain activity monitor being used during your anesthesia.

In 2005, the American Society of Anesthesiologists (ASA) issued their "Practice Advisory for Intraoperative Awareness and Brain Function Monitoring." One of the conclusions of this advisory states: "It is the consensus of the task force that the decision to use a brain function monitor should be made on a case-by-case basis by the individual practitioner for selected patients."

Furthermore, a survey among ASA members asked for a response to the following statement: "Brain function monitors are valuable and should be used to reduce the risk of intraoperative awareness for patients with conditions that may place them at risk for intraoperative awareness." Sixty-nine percent of the ASA members agreed or strongly agreed while only eleven percent of the members disagreed or strongly disagreed with this statement.

According to recent information discussed at the 2007 Annual Meeting of the American Society of Anesthesiologists, the majority of reported cases of awareness under general anesthesia had a muscle paralyzing drug used as part of the anesthetic regimen. For decades a muscle blockade monitor has been available to help assess the level of muscle paralysis when muscle paralyzing drugs are used.

In your pre-operative anesthesia visit, inquire if a muscle relaxant will be used as part of your anesthetic regimen. If the answer is yes, then respectfully request that this monitor be used on you. Furthermore, you can request that at least one twitch remains on the monitor. When no muscle paralysis is present, the monitor will show four twitches. When complete muscle paralysis is present, there will be no twitches on the monitor. In this state, you are completely unable to make any kind of movement in response to a painful stimulus. It is in this state when the anesthetic depth gets too light that a patient can experience awareness under general anesthesia and is unable to make the anesthesia personnel aware that he/she is awake.

Finally, if your surgery can be done safely under some form of local block anesthesia (i.e. spinal, epidural, arm or leg block) with or without intravenous sedation, consider this route. This bypasses general anesthesia and avoids the chances of experiencing awareness under general anesthesia.

REMEMBER: Knowledge is power. Speak up for your rights as a patient!

IN SUMMARY

In your preoperative anesthesia visit, you should discuss . . .

- Your concerns about awareness under anesthesia and receive complete answers to your questions.

- Any problems you have had with previous anesthetics, including past awareness. It is critical that you make anesthesia personnel aware of any prescription drugs or over-the-counter medications you are taking, and how long you have been taking any of these medicines.

- Discuss the use of the brain activity monitor if general anesthesia is to be used and the use of the muscle blockade monitor if a muscle relaxant drug will be used.

- If your surgery can be done safely under some form of local block anesthesia with or without sedation, this bypasses general anesthesia and decreases your chances of experiencing awareness under general anesthesia.

F. W. Ernst, M.D. — William G. Pace III, M. D.

CHAPTER TEN

TO SUE OR NOT TO SUE

Dr. Pace

KEY POINT:

- **In order to assure yourself of the best possible outcome in a medical malpractice lawsuit, you must determine beyond a reasonable doubt whether or not negligence occurred, and you must know how to select the best possible attorney to represent you.**

The little girl looked so cute, perched above her suppertime plate of macaroni and cheese—her favorite!—that her momma couldn't stop hugging her!

"Don't worry, I'll be right there beside you the whole time," Gloria Tice kept telling her 10-year-old daughter, Melanie. "You'll just go to sleep and have some nice dreams—and then when you wake up, I'll be there to read *A Wrinkle in Time* with you. And pretty soon, you'll be feeling a lot better!"

For at least the twentieth time, she hugged the curly-haired little girl at the dinner table beside her. "And then in a few weeks, when you're up and about, we'll be headed straight for Disney World!"

Melanie giggled with delight. She had the sweetest dimples! "Momma, can I bring Jumbo to the hospital?" She held up her toy elephant, her favorite bedtime pal in recent months.

"Of course you can, sweetheart! Now, please eat your macaroni—the doctor told us that you can't have any more food until after the operation. But don't worry, it will all be over by lunchtime tomorrow!"

Melanie nodded, and dug her fork into her bowl with comical determination. What an adorable child! And what a terrible shame that her young life had been touched by so much pain in recent years.

But all of that would be changing now: tomorrow morning, the orthopedic surgeons at the Harbor Hospital complex would be operating on the abnormally curved vertebrae in little Melanie's spine. Led by the well known and supremely confident Chief Surgeon, Dr. Hollis Dale, the surgical team hoped to correct the spinal deformity that had made this little girl's life so difficult in recent years.

It was May 10, 1993, in the Washington, D.C. suburb of Alexandria, Virginia, and Mr. and Mrs. Eldon Tice were waiting eagerly for the surgical procedure that would restore their little sweetheart to a normal life.

Their hopes were high—and why not? Hadn't the breezily confident Dr. Dale virtually guaranteed them that he could work wonders with his scalpel?

Everything about the tall, elegant-looking chief surgeon inspired confidence—from the natty pinstripe suits he wore to the gleaming silver Mercedes he piloted around the streets of tranquil Alexandria. "He's the best in the business," the Tices had been told over and over again. "He's got the hands of a master violinist and the mind of an IBM computer. You can't go wrong with Dr. Dale."

Thank heavens for the miracles of modern surgery! "Finish your milk, sweetheart," Mrs. Tice told her daughter now. "I've got some chocolate pudding with whipped cream for you, and there's a new Disney Special on at eight. Then it's time for beddy-bye. You've got a big day coming tomorrow!"

Three hours later, a contented Melanie was drifting off to sleep, with the dog-eared Jumbo resting snugly against her cheek.

But her mother found sleep much harder to come by. Hour after hour, Gloria Tice lay twisting in her bed, listening to the rumble of distant thunder, while being startled by the occasional flashes of lightning that flickered in the window.

Eldon was awake. He was feeling the anxiety, too.

"Do you think it will be all right, honey?"

He patted her shoulder. "Of course it will, Glo. We've got the best surgeon in the Washington area! Besides, we're not talking about open-heart surgery, here—they're only going to straighten out a few vertebrae. Relax, hon, you need your rest."

But nothing helped. Gloria dozed fitfully, and, when the alarm finally went off at six, she rose to find a cold, gray rain lapping against the windows. A Northeasterner was slamming up the East Coast, and the man on Channel 7 kept saying that the weather was going to be absolutely terrible.

****

They drove to Harbor Hospital through a driving downpour—rain so thick and furious that the windshield wipers could barely keep up.

Dazed, numb with anxiety, Gloria struggled to keep smiling reassuringly at Melanie, as they made their way through the interminable admitting process. But at last they were sitting together in the gleaming Surgical Suites lobby, watching somber-faced nurses and doctors hurry in and out.

"Will it hurt much, Mommy?" Melanie was clutching Jumbo hard.

"Not much, sweetheart," Gloria murmured. "You'll fall right asleep, and when you wake up, you'll feel a little pain. But they'll be giving you shots that will take it away. And don't forget—I'll be there as soon as you wake up, with *A Wrinkle in Time*!"

Melanie grinned—and at that moment Dr. Dale came striding confidently through the swinging metal doors.

"Greetings, one and all!" he boomed. But he was barely looking at the three of them; already, his eyes had dropped to the clipboard in his right hand. "Mrs. Tice . . . can you confirm that Melanie has eaten nothing—no solids or liquids—since dinnertime yesterday?"

Gloria nodded. "She hasn't eaten since six o'clock last night." Suddenly, inexplicably, she was picturing the child eating her plate of macaroni and a sharp pang of sorrow went knifing through her. Almost at the same moment, she caught a whiff of the surgeon's after-shave lotion, a brand she didn't like!

But Dr. Dale was rubbing his hands together briskly now. He was all business. "Everybody all set? Great! Melanie, we're gonna ask you to stretch out on the bed now . . ."

As if by magic, two white-coated attendants had appeared at his elbow: they were pushing along a wheeled bed. Gloria held her breath while they helped the child into the proper position on the bed.

At the last moment, just before they rolled her away, littler Melanie piped, "Bye-bye, Momma!" She waved Jumbo once, and the bed began to roll.

Gloria smiled and waved . . . but she felt the knife-pang again, as she watched the child rolling toward Operating Suite No. 4. She didn't like that smell, didn't like the way things were unfolding here! Was it intuition—or was she simply a big "worry wart," as Melanie always said?

Filled with fear, she sagged against Eldon, who seemed to be holding up all right. But Dr. Dale noticed the moment of terror, and shot them both his famous grin. "Relax, folks!" he sang out, and then waved the clipboard at them. "Everything's under control. I tell ya, it's gonna go like clockwork!"

They sat in a stark, beige-painted waiting room outside Suite No. 4 and watched the clock.

Gloria held Eldon's hand. She could see the fear in his own eyes—and she could see him struggling to hide it, to keep it from her. How she loved him for that! It's only about two hours, honey," he said. He kept rubbing her hand in little circles. "Why don't I go get us a cup of coffee?"

He wandered off toward the big cafeteria on Level Two, and Gloria sat there, staring at the beige-colored walls and biting her upper lip. Would everything go all right? Dr. Dale made everything seem so breezy, so routine—surely that meant there could be no danger?

She bit her lip. She waited.

She had no way of knowing, of course, that on the other side of the swinging metal doors, the "Surgical Wizard" was about to trigger the worst medical tragedy that the authors of this book have ever come across during a combined 65 years of practice.

What happened inside surgical suite No. 4 on May 11, 1993, wasn't just "malpractice": it was probably criminal malpractice.

As an eyewitness—a second physician—who watched the horrifying series of surgical miscues unfold that day at Harbor Hospital later pointed out, the "incredibly careless and reckless" Dr. Hollis Dale "performed in a manner that brought shame upon the entire medical profession"—and then compounded his mistakes by falling into a complete panic, instead of taking the surgical steps that could have prevented disaster.

"What happened that day," explains this medical professional, who worked furiously with several other staffers to try to save Melanie Tice, "was that the surgeon was reckless. There's simply no other way to put it!"

"He didn't take his time, and he wasn't careful enough. He must have figured he was too good ever to make a mistake—that's the kind of ego he had."

But the results were catastrophic.

He accidentally cut the inferior vena cava—which is the main vein that brings blood back from the lower part of the body to the heart. And it was a big enough cut that she started bleeding profusely.

According to this physician, who was standing nearby, the reckless surgeon then compounded the mistake, by failing to "pack the wound and slowly unpack it to find out where the bleeding was, and then suture that area."

In other words, Dr. Dale panicked. Fumbling and stumbling, and constantly changing direction, he wasted precious minutes until all eight of the other medical workers in the room were staring in horror at the extent of the bleeding.

"He wasn't doing what he needed to be doing," remembers the medical staffer. "Instead of localizing it and finding out where the bleeding was coming from, he lost his cool. His dissection"—original scalpel cut through the patient's tissue—"was not a safe, precise dissection, and his follow-up was worse."

The orthopedic specialist who was on hand that day was doing his best to help. But it was no use. Everybody in the room understood that Dr. Dale had gotten into bad trouble. For all eight of the other staffers, what followed was the worst 30 minutes of their professional lives.

While blood "pooled" from the wound, the anesthesiologist and his assistant struggled desperately to replace it fast enough to keep her alive. All too soon, however, they ran out of the blood that had been "typed and crossed" for Melanie, in case of emergency; now they were forced to give her "type-specific but unmatched" blood.

But it was too late. Unable to restore enough blood-volume to keep Melanie's system going, the operating room crew watched in anguish as she "arrested"—her stressed-out heart simply stopped beating.

Forty minutes after the "supremely confident"—and supremely reckless—Dr. Dale had made his first incision, Melanie Tice was dead on the table.

And what followed compounded the tragedy for the Tice family.

While several of the staffers who'd been caught up in the struggle wept openly in a nearby scrub room, an ashen-faced Dr. Hollis Dale stumbled back out to the lobby to confront Melanie's worried parents.

If there was any mercy at all in that moment, it was this: Dr. Dale never had to say a word.

Gloria Tice took one look at his tight, white-lipped face, and burst into tears.

"The moment I saw him walk through those doors, I knew we'd lost Melanie," she would be telling listeners, between sobs, for years to come. "My intuition had been right all along—we should have run away from that surgeon as fast as we could.

"You could see it in his attitude, the breezy way he went about his work. That man's recklessness took away our only child!"

Incredible as it may seem, Melanie's parents never received any recompense in the wake of this utterly egregious incident of medical malpractice.

They were robbed, first, of their daughter and then of their rightful compensation for the loss by a display of anguish on the part of the hospital chief and the surgeon, both of whom insisted that Melanie had expired due to "unavoidable medical complications" during the surgery.

It was the oldest trick in the book: Dr. Dale and the hospital bigshots completely "mystified" Melanie's parents with talk of "hemoglobin depletion" and "sudden spinal-trauma-linked blood pressure decline" . . . and in the end, they managed to convince the dazed and grief-stricken parents that the death had been entirely accidental.

****

Rx: When Should You Sue—And Who Should Represent You?

If you stop and think about it, there were actually two tragedies in the Tice case: the unnecessary death of the child, and the outrageous failure to collect reasonable damage for the malpractice involved.

In order to avoid the latter catastrophe, surgical patients who believe that they or their loved ones may have been injured by medical malpractice should understand two key points:
- First, you need to be able to determine accurately whether medical negligence has actually occurred
- Second, you need to be able to select the very best possible legal representative—and that doesn't mean simply flipping through the Yellow Pages or looking to see what law firms are running the most advertisements on TV!

Before we look at the complex problems of medical/surgical negligence—which center on the question of whether or not a "standard of care" was breached during treatment, resulting in an injury to the patient—let's explore the process of trying to determine whether or not you're entitled to substantial financial damage in a malpractice situation.

First of all, you should understand that it will probably be impossible to mount a medical malpractice suit and follow-through with all of the necessary depositions, transcriptions costs, copying costs, and lawyers' hourly fees for less than $20,000—in many cases, for anything less than $50,000.

Remember, too, that these already high starting numbers can multiply themselves many times over, given half the chance!

In order to begin getting a handle on probable litigation-costs, you must look closely at the way the suit will be conducted.

Although a straight "contingency fee" seems like the easiest method for the plaintiff to employ, it's not unusual for a law firm to require that the plaintiff pay for multiple expenses, including expert evaluations of the case, later depositions, etc.

Obviously, in cases of blatant negligence in which a rapid settlement might be expected without a court appearance—such as the amputation of the wrong leg, in a surgery mishap—a law firm may be willing to pay all expenses up-front and then throughout the trial, if there is one.

Often, however, the most difficult proof for a patient to gather is whether negligence in medical care actually took place. While the family physician may be helpful in making this assessment, it's also true that he or she may very well have been involved in the diagnosis and care. And in my experience, when that happens, there's usually a strong temptation on the part of the doctor to sweep any medical transgressions under the rug.

On the other hand, the "lay" friends and relatives of an alleged malpractice victim usually tend to sympathize so much with their pal that they can hardly be objective about negligence. This difficult problem of "biased" assessment cannot be easily solved.

At the same time, the selection of your lawyer is also extremely important. Would you choose a knee surgeon to help you with an infection in your left eye? Of course not! Unfortunately, however, finding a good attorney may not be as simple as merely making sure that the lawyer you select is experienced in malpractice law.

To explain why that's true, let me speak quite bluntly. As a veteran physician, many of my colleagues and I have been harassed for years by a small group of attorneys who will pursue any case, regardless of whether or not it involves actual negligence. One reason is the poor advice they frequently get from so-called "medical experts." I have often read the opinions of "professional experts" who charge exorbitant fees for their assessments and declare a case to be "very litigious"—even when it's obviously the kind of case that would quickly be lost in court.

Let's not pretend about this: the motivation of the "professional witness" is money. And don't forget: if a case is determined to be unworthy of a lawsuit, the expert will receive a single fee; but if the matter can be prolonged through several depositions, that same expert stands to receive additional thousands of dollars. Of course, if the case actually winds up in the courtroom, the same expert stands to make a real killing.

As you might expect in this field, there are some attorneys who also hold medical degrees. And yes, those individuals do frequently have more insight into whether negligence has occurred. But an M.D degree is no guarantee that a lawyer will prove to be as sharp and skilled as the defendant's lawyer!

Most of the defense lawyers against whose clients I have testified have been employed by large insurance companies. These specialists do nothing but malpractice defense and are fairly well educated in medical matters. They are also well supplied with "trick questions" for the plaintiff's expert witness, and are totally ruthless in trying to paint the expert as a professional who will testify to anything for the money, precisely in order to minimize the impact of his or her testimony on the judge and jury.

The jury will always hear two opposite opinions presented by the plaintiff's and the defendant doctor's expert witnesses, and the jurors will have to decide just who is telling the truth: the friends and/or colleagues supporting the defendant doctor or the expert for the plaintiff—who could indeed be a member of the profession, but who in this case is testifying to things that simply aren't true!

How can society arrive at a malpractice verdict that's fair to all concerned?

There is no easy solution. However, I have found that the best justice has not been served by the jury system, but by the federal system which is invoked in the event of malpractice against a veterans' hospital or other federal facility.

Why? Simple: In those cases, a federal judge listens to the evidence from both sides, and decides not only the verdict, but also the size of the award.

A second approach, based on presenting the facts to a "triumvirate" consisting of a doctor, a judge, and a lawyer, has also been employed frequently in this country, but unfortunately, the opinions and recommendations that emerge from this method of jurisprudence aren't binding in most cases, and can still be carried on to trial.

Although I have often seen this system fail—usually because a doctor has voted for his colleague, even in the face of gross negligence—it seems the fairest method, overall, and usually avoids the recommendations for exorbitant awards that are often made by juries.

Still, I don't think it's fair to burden the average jury with the medical jargon—that requires a full year of study on the part of the average medical student—to say nothing of the task of understanding the "nuances" of the art and science of surgery, or the difficult problem of understanding the factual basis for "absolute standards of care."

Of course, most attorneys who specialize in medical malpractice are usually well-informed on medicine and deviations from standards of care. He or she will often employ a retired nurse to assist in the preliminary review of a patient's claim before even requesting a copy of a chart from a hospital—because that is where the real expenses begin.

Once that chart has been ordered and received, you can be sure that many hours of grueling work lie ahead.

And you should be forewarned: In my experience, it's not uncommon for a hospital not only to charge exorbitantly for a copy of these records, but also to "conveniently" scramble them, thus adding many hours of sorting time for the lawyer's assistant or the expert who will review them eventually and recommend a course of action to the lawyer.

Take note: almost fifty percent of the cases I'm asked to review don't actually represent negligence, but only a misunderstanding between doctor and patient.

All too often, as it turns out, an unsympathetic or "too busy" doctor manages to evade being tagged with actual negligence, even though his cold-blooded aloofness certainly demands at least a reprimand. And yet these violators usually escape, after the plaintiff's attorneys conclude that outright negligence probably can't be proved in the courtroom, and then convince their clients to drop the suits.

Interestingly, however, the plaintiffs in two cases that I worked on refused to be so dissuaded, and went on to select new attorneys and to proceed with their lawsuits. (In both of those cases, the defendants subsequently retained me as an expert witness, and then prevailed.)

Next question: Is a lawsuit always necessary in cases of alleged malpractice?

Answer: Absolutely not—and it should not happen, except as a last resort. A lawsuit is a devastating experience for the defendant physician. But if he's caring, compassionate, and kind in dealing with the patient and the patient's family, such suits will often be nipped in the bud.

More than once, I've removed sponges from patients who were referred to me by surgeons from outside small communities, and, in every case, I was pleasantly surprised when the patient and family understood, respected, and trusted the local doctor, regardless of the miscue, and refused to file a lawsuit.

My favorite true story of this kind involved a dear friend who was also a well-known football coach. We both came to Ohio State in the 1950s, and, when he had his gallbladder removed by a colleague of mine, a sponge was left behind. The coach became very ill, toxic, and he nearly died before the sponge was at last removed without further incident.

In the past, of course, such a misstep had been considered the basis for an indefensible lawsuit. At the time of the coach's discharge, however, as the surgeon was apologizing profusely, the old coach flung an arm around him and barked, "Stop it, son. Forget it! I'm the only one who never made a mistake!"

Were we surprised by this sudden forgiveness? Not those of us who knew the accident victim as one of the greatest gentlemen of our era, or his former players, most of whom continue to worship him even today.

Do mistakes occur in surgery? Of course they do, as much as surgeons might like to pretend otherwise. I don't deny that I've made a few errors that would certainly be considered deviations from standards of care, or negligence. But I was careful to discuss these mistakes later with those few patients, and thankfully, they never opted for a lawsuit. And while openness won't solve every problem, trying to cover it up or deny it usually does fuel the fire of a potential lawsuit.

Also: while admission of guilt or wrongdoing by the defendant surgeon may not be accepted as a signal to pay a claim by his insurance carrier, it seems clear to me that if such a policy could be followed, we'd see far less medical litigation than we do today.

Is it really possible to find ways to minimize the possibility of a mistake in any given surgical procedure? That is indeed the "$64,000 Question!" There's an old saying about patients in this country, which points out that they have a lot of choices in selecting a physician: they can pick the first one! And that's true to a certain degree.

Example: A number of years ago, a young lady visited my office and asked me to perform her gallbladder surgery. We scheduled the surgery for later in the week. But then, surprisingly, she showed up at my office again. She cried as she told me how, when she'd informed her family physician that she'd asked me to do the cholecystectomy, he called her into his office, reviewed her charts and records for half an hour, and then announced that if she insisted on going to me, he would no longer take care of her! And although this particular doctor has now passed on to his greater reward, I'm afraid that such behavior still occurs all too frequently in the medical community. There's no question that doctors have certain referral patterns, and that they attempt to direct patients accordingly.

The motivation behind these referrals is rather obvious: "You scratch my back and I'll scratch yours." Yes, I've had many patients tell me that their family physicians became furious when they asked to be referred to the Mayo Clinic for a second opinion. My solution to that would be simply to find another family physician.

Years ago, of course, the medical profession was damaged terribly by the practice of "fee splitting," in which a surgeon would rebate part of the surgical fee in return for a referral. That practice is illegal—and regarded as unethical—but a last vestige remains, via the employment of non-surgical referring physicians as assistants in the operating room, where they will "hold retractors" or otherwise "assist"— while collecting a separate fee. If that arrangement becomes frequent between a family physician and his favorite surgeon to whom he refers surgical cases, it's easy enough to understand why a family physician or internist would be reluctant to refer a case to a surgeon requested by the patient!

Yet it's the patient's right to know about these arrangements, and the answer can only be learned by asking. Let's face it: A family physician or internist rarely has been trained adequately in surgery, and, personally, I don't want him or her in the operating room—especially if I'm going to be paying the fee!

No, if I'm going to pay a fee to an assistant, I want to meet him or her, and to discuss my case, while learning about that person's training and background. I also would like to discuss the need for this paid assistant with my surgeon. Of course, there are indeed occasional problems in surgery that mandate the presence of another specialist who will require a fee: A prime example would be surgery involving a related-donor kidney transplant, where one surgeon safely harvests and handles the healthy kidney without injury to the donor, while the other one removes the diseased kidney and replaces it.

For the majority of routine procedures, however, a second paid assistant is simply "pocketbook padding," and it's the right of the patient to know all the details!

Remember, too, that "informed consent" is one of the most important components of an operation. The patient should pay close attention, ask many questions, and demand straight answers during this process—even to the point of taking notes. Why? Well, for one thing, extensive research has shown that when patients were asked for informed consent by their surgeons, and the sessions were tape-recorded, the patients later denied having given such consent to 40 percent of the procedures to which they had consented on the tape!

Other studies show an even greater discrepancy. How could this happen? The answer can be found in the dialogue that takes place between patient and doctor, during this period of extreme stress prior to anesthesia and surgery. Don't forget that informed consent, which covers every surgical eventuality, must be signed in the presence of a nurse or admitting clerk. All too often, it's the only evidence on the chart that the patient was told what kind of surgery was noted in the space marked "fill in the name of operation on the blank line."

Finally, let's talk about two other types of surgical procedures that demand the close scrutiny of the patient: exploratory laparotomy and exploratory surgery. These two procedures are both vague at best. What, exactly, is an exploratory laparotomy? Truthfully, even though I've done some of them, I'm not sure I know! All too often, it's the last medical refuge, after a patient has been complaining of indefinable pains for a long time, and the family physician has finally reached the "limit of tolerance."

Make no mistake: A patient who is about to undergo an exploratory laparotomy should be extremely inquisitive about specific indications, percentages, expectations, and, most importantly, exactly what the surgery is expected to accomplish. (A second and even a third opinion is in order and should be demanded.)

Quire frankly, the overall yield on an exploratory laparotomy is as close to zero as anything in medicine. If the operation is done to relieve pain alone, the results will usually be miserable for anything more than "adhesions." And although patients will often improve temporarily after the surgery for reasons that we don't fully understand, the source of the pain will usually erupt again within a few weeks.

On the other hand, we do know that millions of patients with extensive adhesions are out there walking around without pain, and that there's simply no physiological explanation for adhesions causing anything more serious than rare intestinal obstruction—which is a very typical pain complex, and demands exploration under most circumstances. I learned in medical school what millions of other doctors have learned: "Confucius say, 'He who operate on pain will not find it'," and I think that maxim still applies today.

Of course, the prospects for finding the cause of "fever of undetermined origin" aren't much better! In this medical nightmare, the patient suffers daily—or even twice daily—from spikes of fever, but without any apparent infection. What's going on here? It's hard to say; some of these cases remain a mystery, even after thorough study.

It's possible that an occult malignancy might be responsible—a possibility that may, indeed, justify an exploratory laparotomy. Another treatable source for the fever may be in the abdomen. And, indeed, an exploratory laparotomy designed to discover the nature of a mass identified during a physical exam—or through a scan in some other diagnostic method—seems almost certain to produce positive results. Still, it's necessary for patients to clarify absolutely what will be removed at the time of this exploratory surgery.

REMEMBER: Always demand answers (and even second opinions), so that you can avoid later surprises, as well as recriminations!

IN SUMMARY

- In order to assure yourself of the best possible outcome in a medical malpractice lawsuit, you must determine beyond a reasonable doubt whether or not "negligence" occurred, and you must know how to select the best possible attorney to represent you.

- After concluding that you've been a victim of medical malpractice, use the steps in this chapter to find the legal specialist who's exactly right for your particular case. Forget the Yellow Pages—do some research!

- There are several methods used for adjudicating malpractice cases in the U. S. (jury, "triumvirate" and single judge), but the best system is the one in which the case is both heard and decided by a single judge.

F. W. Ernst, M.D. — William G. Pace III, M. D.

CHAPTER ELEVEN

MALPRACTICE OPTIONS

Dr. Pace

KEY POINT:

- **Whether the case is heard by a jury, a single judge, or a mandatory arbitration panel, the danger of an unfair verdict cannot be eliminated.**

Make no mistake: what you don't know about surgery and anesthesia can kill you. Thankfully, it doesn't happen very often. But when the delicate process of administering general anesthesia and then performing surgery goes awry, the results can be tragic and horrifying.

They can also trigger some amazingly complicated "malpractice cases," extraordinary legal battles in which plaintiffs and defendants slug it out for years at a time in the vast and swarming labyrinth that is the U.S. court system.

As you might imagine, there have been endless efforts over the years to find the "perfect method" for trying medical malpractice lawsuits, a method that would protect the rights of all, while at the same time guaranteeing a fair and equitable verdict in each and every case.

Unfortunately, however, there appears to be no such method; each of the various systems for adjudicating malpractice lawsuits (jury trial, single judge, mandatory arbitration before a tribunal, etc.) has the potential—if things go wrong in the courtroom—to produce a horrendous miscarriage of justice.

F. W. Ernst, M.D. — William G. Pace III, M. D.

And that's exactly what happened in the tiny, Ohio farm town of Collington, back in the mid-1990s, when a bouncy, fun-loving college student named Mandy paid the ultimate price for an anesthetist's mistake.

After being assigned to review the extraordinary malpractice case that resulted from this tragic incident, I found myself asking the same terrible question over and over again: How could a trained professional have allowed this disaster to happen?

As you're about to discover, the ghastly story of what happened to Mandy Carter speaks volumes about the dangers of surgical anesthesia, and also about the deeply troubling flaws in the American system for litigating malpractice lawsuits, whether that system is based on trial by jury, trial by judge, or arguments before an arbitration panel.

Before we take a look at the strengths and weaknesses of the various methods for litigating malpractice, however, we need to understand the human dimensions of such cases. We need to experience—up close and personal—some of the agony that Mandy and other victims of malpractice must endure, when things go wrong in the operating room.

For Mandy Carter of Collington, Ohio, the tragedy began harmlessly enough with an occasional flash of mild pain in her lower abdomen. Nothing major. Just a quick, stabbing sensation down there below her tummy . . . then gone.

Sitting on the big leather sofa in her mother's handsomely furnished living room, 19-year-old Mandy frowned and shook her head. "Hey, Mom . . . I think I'm getting some kind of stomach ache. Maybe it's that pepperoni pizza we had at the bowling alley!"

Wiping her hands on her bright yellow apron, Mrs. Florence Carter stepped into the living room. "I hope you're not getting the flu, honey—it seems like everybody in town has been hit, lately. Do you have a fever?"

Lovingly, she patted her only daughter's forehead.

It was Saturday afternoon, about five o'clock, in the south Ohio farming settlement of Collington, located about 70 miles east of Athens. Home from Kent State University for the weekend, the hard-charging history major with the blonde pony-tail had spent the afternoon at a duckpin bowling lane in nearby Brewerton, accompanied by her two favorite cousins, Chad and Chris.

Now, stretched out on the sofa in the family's big stone farmhouse on rural Route 3, Mandy kept complaining about her worsening "stomach ache". And, yes . . . she did seem to be running a bit of fever, about 100 degrees, with occasional chills. . .

As the hours passed, Mandy got sicker.

Unable to join her family at the dinner table, she lay immobile in the living room, trying not to think about the ever-increasing misery that her body was putting her through.

By eleven, the pain was so bad that Mandy was in tears. Hugging her mid-section, she rocked back and forth on the sofa . . . while her mother paced about, increasingly fretful. Mandy's temperature was now 102°—although there had been no nausea, no vomiting so far. If this were a routine case of intestinal flu, why wasn't she nauseated?

At one a.m., with Mandy weeping helplessly and her swollen abdomen "hard as a rock," Mrs. Carter decided it was time to act. Quickly she dialed the emergency room at the small Willerton County Hospital, about ten miles distant. "Could it be appendicitis?" she asked the nurse on duty.

The nurse thought so, and so did the general practitioner M.D (we'll call him "Dr. GP") who was running the Emergency Room that night.

"Looks like acute appendicitis," Dr. GP told Mandy's troubled Mom, after running a few tests. "All of the classical symptoms are present—intense pain in the lower right abdomen, along with fever, swelling, tenderness."

Mrs. Carter nodded helplessly.

"The danger right now is peritonitis," said the doctor, as he scribbled something on a clipboard. "We must go in right now and take care of it—the surgical team will be ready in 25 minutes. You'll have to sign a release. . ."

Mrs. Carter's hand shook noticeably as she scrawled her name on the paper.

When she looked up, Dr. GP was standing beside her again. "Mrs. Carter, Mandy tells me that she hasn't eaten anything since noontime. True?"

The worried mother rushed to confirm this, "Yes—she skipped dinner entirely. She went bowling with her cousins, around noon, and they all had pizza. And I'm certain that she hasn't eaten since."

"I see." The doctor scribbled on his clipboard again.

And it was here that the first link in the chain of tragedy would be formed—as Dr. GP foolishly accepted Mandy's and Mrs. Carter's description of her food intake that day. In fact, both mother and daughter were wrong. Feverish and groaning with pain, the distracted Mandy had harped on the fact that she'd "missed dinner" . . . without pointing out that she'd actually consumed a large slice of pizza and most of a chocolate milkshake around 4 p.m., just before the end of the bowling session with her cousins.

Of course, Mandy's mother only compounded the mistake, by frantically insisting, "She hasn't eaten since the middle of the day—when she had pizza."

That was the first link in the terrible chain.

The second one was forged only a few minutes later, when Dr. GP inexplicably failed to remember a basic fact about the hazards of peritonitis: when that condition is impending, the stomach cannot and will not empty itself, except via the esophagus and mouth, through vomiting.

But Mandy had not yet been stricken with any vomiting.

While considering this fact, Dr. GP next failed—for reasons that remain unclear to this day—to take an absolutely crucial step in preparing any patient for pre-operative, general anesthesia: he failed to eliminate the danger of a discharge of stomach contents by presuming that the patient had a full stomach—regardless of what she or anybody else said.

In other words, Dr. GP instructed his Certified Registered Nurse Anesthetist (CRNA) to administer general anesthesia without the benefit of an endotracheal tube, a "breathing tube" inserted into the trachea to ensure an unobstructed airflow during surgery.

Because this rural hospital was too small to employ its own anesthesiologist, Dr. GP was forced to rely on the skill and experience of the CRNA, who also apparently failed to consider the possibility of performing an 'awake intubation," a safe procedure in which the "breathing tube" can be inserted with the patient still conscious, in order to protect against a dangerous discharge during anesthesia-induced unconsciousness.

Unbelievably, given the patient's symptoms, the befuddled physician also decided to proceed without a stomach-evacuation tube of any sort.

The results were as predictable as they were tragic: as soon as Mandy's body relaxed under the general anesthetic, the sphincter (or controlling muscle at the top of the stomach, where it joins the esophagus) also relaxed—triggering a nightmarish scenario in which her stomach contents, mostly still undigested, flowed swiftly up the esophagus and into the trachea.

During the next few terrible minutes, Mandy Carter drowned in her own gastric content.

By then, of course, Dr. GP was utterly powerless to undo the chain of disaster that his mistakes had forged. Because he'd taken the hazy statements of his patient and her mother as fact—while failing to defend against the obvious danger of a stomach-discharge—Dr. GP had thoughtlessly triggered the "drowning" of his own surgical patient, via the general anesthetic.

By the time the surgeon discovered Mandy to be suffering from a perforation of a cecal diverticulum—in fact, the young woman's appendix was normal—it didn't matter: tragically, the young woman lay pulseless on the operating table.

How heartbreaking it must have been for Florence Carter to listen to the testimony during the malpractice trial that took place a few years later, and to read a hospital report in which the fumbling "Dr. GP" described how he had insisted on "finishing the operation and sewing up the patient"…before sending the youthful Mandy Carter on to the funeral home.

To this day, the ghastly story of how Mandy Carter's life was snuffed out by a careless application of anesthesia remains one of the most horrifying cases of malpractice.

However, this terrible story didn't end with the young college student's death. The extraordinary, five-year battle that followed in the courts—a $2 million extravaganza that ultimately required the services of 17 lawyers and produced 117,000 pages of testimony and related documents—also wound up as a major tragedy for Mrs. Carter and her grieving family.

Astonishingly, in what may be the single greatest miscarriage of justice that this physician experienced during a career spent reviewing such litigation (usually as an "expert witness"), Mandy Carter's family received only the limit of the doctor's insurance, a minuscule $100,000—of which at least $50,000 was eaten up by legal fees and other costs.

In the end, the Carter family received nothing more than what the lawyers call "chump change" for the agonizing tragedy that Dr. GP's obvious negligence had inflicted on them.

Incredible, also, was this startling fact: the jury actually allowed the doctor to continue practicing medicine!

How, exactly, did this jury trial of the doctor's "peers" produce such a grotesquely unjust verdict?

To answer that question, we must step back for a moment and take a brief look at the three basic methods now used in the United States to litigate malpractice cases.

****

Rx: No matter what form the litigation takes, the key to a fair verdict is always a thorough presentation of the facts.

The most common method, and the one which is probably most familiar to lay people in this country, is the jury trial, in which a jury of the defendant medical professional's peers must evaluate the evidence and then decide whether or not malpractice did, indeed, occur.

Of course, the major difficulty in this form of jurisprudence is the difficulty of "educating" a group of ordinary citizens about medical issues and procedures—some of which will inevitably be quite complex and intellectually challenging.

One way around that dilemma is to allow such malpractice cases to be heard by a single judge, without a jury, providing that both sides agree to this formula. But this form of litigation can present some extraordinary problems of its own, as I learned the hard way, while serving as an "expert witness" many years ago during one of my first malpractice cases.

F. W. Ernst, M.D. — William G. Pace III, M. D.

The whole thing began rather oddly, when I was sent a case from Jamaica through the mail—along with a check to pay for a review of the entire litigation. The Jamaican lawyer didn't ask about my fee, or whether his check was adequate—indeed, I didn't even know how his law firm had obtained my name!

But I quickly became fascinated by the facts of this unusual case, in which a young mother had been operated on for a cholecystectomy, or removal of the gall bladder. Her medical chart—nearly six inches thick—showed that the surgery had been performed by a local practitioner who noted in the record that a "cholangiogram" had been necessary at the time of surgery, because of multiple small stones.

Unfortunately, however, he had failed to do the cholangiogram, a fact which became especially troubling after this operation when the patient developed jaundice and massive fluid in the abdomen. While the surgeon went on vacation, his assistant invested thousands of dollars in studies aimed at uncovering the cause of the young woman's jaundice. But when these failed to explain the ailment, he took matters into his own hands and performed a choledochojejunostomy, an operation in which the surgeon connects the bile duct directly to the intestine.

Usually, of course, this type of operation is reserved for cases in which there has been an injury to the bile duct system at the time of the first surgery.

Strangely enough, the findings at the time of the second surgery were completely omitted from the operation notes, a fact which convinced the plaintiff's attorney that the assistant was covertly attempting to protect his boss.

The trial that followed was unique. It was presided over by a federal judge, with no jury present. A specially appointed interpreter was assigned to translate for me. As you might imagine, I was quite curious to discover why I had been "imported" from Ohio. And the explanation soon emerged: it seemed that the father of the defendant was a very powerful man, that his mother was an important lawyer on the local scene, and that his sister was a district attorney. In short, no local "expert witness" wanted to come within a hundred miles of that case!

Another unusual legal twist occurred when the judge, having received a copy of the letter I'd sent to the plaintiff's lawyers, concluded in advance that the defendant doctor would lose the case; as a result, he advised the lady lawyer for the defendant to settle. (She refused, however, while insisting that the plaintiffs wanted too much money.)

As the case progressed, I found myself patiently explaining to the judge that the bile ducts had surely been injured at some point, but that the disappearance of the operative notes made it impossible to determine whether the damage had been done during the initial procedure, or later during the assistant's "repair" procedure. Still, there was no doubt that negligence had occurred.

I also emphasized the fact that if stones had been left behind to cause the blockage and the jaundice (after the first procedure), thus triggering the rupture of the bile duct because of the pressure of the bile fluid in the biliary tract, then the proper medical care would have been to simply remove the stones, place a tube in the bile duct, and close the patient.

Under no circumstances whatsoever should the poor woman's bile duct have been sewn to the intestines, as had occurred in this case.

It was an extraordinary experience. After three days on the witness stand in a 100-degree courtroom, I suddenly discovered an extremely revealing drawing in the thousands of pages of the official record. Quickly, I interrupted the judge and explained to him that this document had been omitted from the records which I had received.

That drawing was quite revealing, and it had obviously been executed by a person who was both medically knowledgeable and artistically gifted. It showed a bile duct and a gallbladder, with a line drawn through the connection with the bile duct, showing where the gallbladder had been removed. And two round objects—clearly visible and obviously stones—had been drawn in the remaining bile duct!

I rapidly pointed out to the judge that this drawing proved a critical point: Although two stones were present instead of just one, the surgical problem was nonetheless quite easy to solve—and without even the slightest damage to the bile ducts. (I also noted for the record that the second operation had been negligently performed as well.)

Late in the third day of the trial, the defense lawyer made the fatal mistake of asking questions without already knowing the answers, when she began to ask me about board certification exams in an obvious bid to undermine my creditability.

Although I knew nothing about the "board certification status" of the defendant doctor, I quickly pointed out that there was a 30% failure rate in these exams.

Surprised, she blurted: "Of all candidates?"

"No," I replied. "In the United States, we have a class of doctors who cannot get into American medical schools and are sent by their rich daddies to Guadalajara. Probably 100% of that group fail their exams."

Instantly, the courtroom erupted, as the young mother screamed and had to be removed from the proceedings by the bailiff. The defendant doctor was also roaring and hollering, and could only be silenced by the judge's threat to hold him in contempt.

Even the defendant's lawyer—who had opened this Pandora's box in the first place—had to be restrained from howling her lungs out!

The plaintiff's lawyers roared with laughter, and only then did I discover that the defendant had not been able to get into an American medical school, and had indeed been sent by his wealthy and prominent father to Guadalajara . . . and that he had subsequently failed his board exams.

As you might expect, the judge ruled for the plaintiff (although the amount of the settlement had to be determined at another trial). This case is a good example of the justice that can be delivered by a judge without a jury.

Another method that has been tried in many states has been "mandatory arbitration" before a tribunal consisting of a judge, a lawyer for the defendant doctor, and another physician.

My own limited experience with this approach has taught me that there are both good and bad aspects, starting, first of all, with the troublesome question of whether or not such litigation violates the defendant's right to a trial by a jury of one's peers.

It's actually quite impossible to gather a jury of peers when the defendant is a medical doctor. Why? Well, it's pretty unlikely that a panel of twelve unbiased physicians could be rounded up for such a jury, and, even if they were, each one could expect to be sternly challenged for his seat by the defense.

Another problem with the arbitration system is that, if both sides don't approve of the outcome, the case will go to trial anyway.

Also troubling, here, is the fact that the physician on the tribunal maintains a veto power, a state of affairs which can result in a negative verdict that's very unfair to the injured patient, even in the case of clearly demonstrable negligence.

That's precisely what happened to Mandy Carter's family, in the tragic story that began this chapter. After she drowned in her own fluids in the operating room of that rural hospital in Ohio, you will recall, her family received a paltry award of $100,000 (the limit of the doctor's liability insurance) for the loss of her life through his inexcusable negligence.

That thoroughly unjust verdict occurred because of the great weakness of the tribunal system of litigation, which gave the other physician on the panel veto-power over the proceedings and allowed him to cheat Mandy Carter's heirs out of damages they clearly deserved.

Of course, that extraordinarily unfair settlement also allowed "Dr. GP" to go right on practicing medicine. And what was the result? He promptly became involved in yet another egregious case of malpractice.

Dr. GP's second fiasco centered on a 40-year-old man whom the doctor had treated for a rash on his penis with a cortisone cream for six months.

The gentleman was uncircumcised, and, although the doctor testified before the trial tribunal that he had tried repeatedly to convince the man to undergo a circumcision, there was no record of such a conversation, or of a refusal.

Eventually, however, the circumcision was performed, and the foreskin was forwarded to a local pathologist, who became quite concerned about the specimen.

This specialist made a tentative diagnosis of "erythroplasia of Queyrat," a benign condition. (His notes described a one-centimeter-elevated lesion with a punctuate center at the edge of the specimen.)

The pathologist was so concerned that he sent the specimen off to a university for a final diagnosis. The report came back with the shocking disclosure that this was, indeed, an invasive carcinoma of the skin of the penis. Since this is a condition found only in uncircumcised males, it should have been suspected by the doctor—especially given the elevated lesion on the skin which was "close to the edge" where he had cut off the foreskin.

The lawyer who brought this case to me pointed out that the defendant doctor had nearly gone into shock when he discovered this report in his files after the lawsuit had been filed—and realized that he had overlooked it while treating the patient.

Still, the failure to read the report wasn't the only negligence taking place here: the doctor merely contented himself with examining the patient during the next several months; his records did not indicate that he had ever again referred to the problems at the site of the penis.

Finally, months later, the patient returned to his office to complain of itching of the penis, and was again treated with cortisone cream, but apparently without the doctor referring to the past medical records that were available to him.

Later still, with the situation continuing to deteriorate, the patient's girlfriend insisted that he consult a urologist, who confirmed the diagnosis of recurrent cancer, which was now so advanced that it would require amputation of the penis.

The trial in this case also took place before a tribunal. First the defense attempted to discredit me as a witness, after which the defendant's lawyer insisted that, even if the diagnosis had been made earlier, the patient would have still lost his penis! (According to the defense's truly amazing line of argument, the patient was actually better off because of the failure-to-diagnose—after all, he'd had the use of his penis for several extra months, hadn't he?)

As in the earlier case, the verdict here was for the plaintiff, but only for the limit of the insurance, in a settlement that was agreed to by the defense. But it's hard to believe that a jury would have been so forgiving in deciding how best to compensate that unfortunate young man.

My only other encounter with an arbitration panel was even less pleasant, mainly because of the presence on the panel of a physician who had decided, in advance of hearing the evidence, that he would not support a finding of negligence under any circumstances. His unreasonable, negative vote triggered a split two-to-one vote, and thus wasted a great deal of money.

In this case, the dispute centered on an operation in which the defendant doctor had completely cut across the common bile duct during a gallbladder operation while using the laparoscopic technique. The operating surgeon had actually encountered many difficulties during the procedure, but had decided to continue, rather than opening the abdomen and completing the operation under direct vision. As a result, the patient was returned to a room and allowed to develop severe peritonitis before a reparative operation was finally accomplished.

In an arbitration proceeding, the situation is somewhat similar to a courtroom trial—but without a jury and usually without all of the grandstanding tricks that characterize the behavior of defense attorneys when performing before a jury. In this case the physician-member of the panel simply assumed the attitude that malpractice did not exist. And that kind of closed-mindedness is the basic problem with all of these physician-developed arbitration systems.

In this particular case, the split decision meant that the defendants settled the case for $150,000, rather than risking a jury trial. (Such an outcome is no proof of anything, of course, because nobody can predict what a jury might do or the size of an award it might grant. But the outcome does underline the fact that the physician-member of that jury was less than objective, so that any potential benefits of the panel system in that case were completely negated!)

If we compare the methods of adjudicating malpractice claims today to a shopping experience in which the shopper has a choice between merely "good," "better" or "best," then it's obvious that the best option of all is simply to let the judge decide cases alone. The next best option is the arbitration panel, while the jury system rapidly plunges us into the area of the unknown—and all too often, the ridiculous.

The only objective lesson that I've learned over the past 25 years is that a doctor who is absolutely and unquestionably guilty should request a jury trial and a good lawyer.

Although there are many exceptions and all juries are not the same, it's true that jury trials tend to differ, based on locale. For instance, juries in large cities tend more to be "free and easy" with what they assume is the insurance company's money, even if a physician is uninsured.

Truth, Lies and the OR

The smaller the town, meanwhile, the greater the tendency is to find in favor of the local doctor—especially if the "imported experts" are testifying for the plaintiff. And there's also the problem of association with the local doctor—who in one case I worked had operated on everyone in the courtroom, including all of the jury and even the judge! It's hardly possible to hope for an honest verdict in that environment.

Perhaps the best courtroom environment of all—at least for victims of malpractice—is the inner city in a large urban area. Such a setting was the backdrop for one of my first devastating experiences in malpractice litigation. This case appeared to be as much of a "sure thing" as you could hope for—yet it was lost.

Here the jury was predominantly inner-city and African-American, while the defendant doctor was a Caucasian. The plaintiff, an African-American, had triggered this comedy of errors when he sought advice about leg cramps, which struck whenever he walked more than a block. Since he was a heavy smoker, the proper action—regardless of angiograms or X-rays of blood vessels of the extremity—was to insist that he quit the smoking and begin an exercise program. By following those guidelines, many patients will re-establish blood flow to the legs, and thus escape surgery. (As a matter of fact, during the days when I was doing peripheral vascular surgery, I would not operate on a patient who refused to give up the cigarettes.)

This particular patient was examined with an angiogram. The doctor read it, and informed the patient that he needed surgery on his right leg, a procedure calling for a bypass from the main blood vessel, the aorta, to the femoral artery, the artery to the distal leg. So far, so good: the patient agreed and was admitted to the hospital. The following day—with the patient still smoking—the bypass was accomplished. Then, without obtaining informed consent, and simply on the basis of "feeling" the other side, the doctor proceeded to do a bypass on the left side as well!

F. W. Ernst, M.D. — William G. Pace III, M. D.

In the recovery room after surgery both distal legs became blue, and the pulses disappeared or became weak (the charts seem confused). No Doppler measurements were taken. (A Doppler is a small instrument which looks like a stainless-steel ball-point pen, with one square end and a wire emerging from the other end to connect with a black box containing electronics, batteries and a small speaker. When the instrument is placed over a vessel, even in the absence of a pulse, a whoosh can be heard, indicating that there is indeed a pulsatile blood flow, even if it can't be felt.)

No such instrument was used in this case, however, and the defendant doctor insisted that none had been available, even though in terms of contemporary medicine, such failure to keep one on hand would clearly constitute deviation from proper standards of care.

Now, it should be understood that when the pulses become weak after a bypass, the reason is almost invariably a technical problem, caused either by the suture of the blood vessels or by what is referred to as "trash foot," a situation in which the lining of the vessel becomes so diseased that particles of cholesterol and calcium break off and travel down the bloodstream, thereby plugging the vessels.

And the only acceptable treatment is to restore the blood flow by taking the patient back to the operating room and inserting a tiny catheter or tube with a small balloon at the end (called a Fogarty catheter) down the artery as far as possible, then inflating the balloon and pulling it back, thus removing the particles and clots that plug the tiny distal arteries.

An X-ray may or may not be taken at this time, but this maneuver usually restores the blood flow, and the trauma to the patient is minimal. In this case, however, nothing was done. The surgeon made a diagnosis of acute venous inflammation, or phlebitis, which is never seen this rapidly after an operation on the leg arteries. With the doctor declining to re-explore the arteries to correct the situation, he and his staff stood by and watched gangrene develop... to the point that both legs were eventually amputated.

It was an incredible case of negligence. First, there was the unnecessary surgery. Next, surgery without informed consent had been performed on the uninvolved leg. Third, the doctor had failed to remove the clots post-operatively, or to save the legs. Finally, the doctor made an incorrect diagnosis of thrombophlebitis, which never causes gangrene, and which was shown not to be present at all in either of the removed legs, when they were examined in the lab.

In spite of the immense weight of all this evidence and testimony, however, the jury found the defendant not guilty of negligence. Why? The reasons they gave came down to their belief that "this was just a 70-year-old man who would have probably lost his legs sooner or later, anyway!"

Furthermore, they seemed convinced that a "big-time" vascular surgeon like this one couldn't make mistakes of this sort—after all, wasn't this minor surgery for a genius like him? This case proved that juries are unpredictable, to say the least.

These cases all illustrate the complicated problems that are inherent in all malpractice actions. And, while a jury trial may represent the least favorable option, it should be pointed out that not all juries are the same. In reality, a tribunal that includes members with preconceived notions and prejudices may not manage to deliver a fairer verdict than the one handed down by a "jury of one's peers."

The best approach, in my opinion, is simply to conduct malpractice cases before a single judge. But always remember: whatever the method of adjudication, no malpractice case is ever a sure thing!

F. W. Ernst, M.D. — William G. Pace III, M. D.

IN SUMMARY

- Whether the malpractice case is heard by a jury, a single judge, or a mandatory arbitration panel, the danger of an unfair verdict cannot be eliminated.

- No matter what form the litigation takes, the best chance for a fair verdict will always depend on a clear, simple presentation of the facts.

In jury trials, the great challenge confronting the attorneys on both sides is trying to educate the jury by presenting enormously complex medical information clearly and succinctly.

CHAPTER TWELVE

LESSONS FOR EVERYONE:
What We Can Learn from Unsuccessful Malpractice Cases

Dr. Pace

KEY POINT:

- **Surgical patients and other health-care consumers can protect themselves against medical negligence quite effectively by taking the trouble to understand why so many malpractice cases end in defeat for the plaintiffs—even though the complaining patients were, indeed, injured by incompetent physicians.**

Years later, long after the horror of the botched operation, and long after the equally botched malpractice trial, Jenny Kramer would remember the moment when it all began: the moment when she first felt a lump.

"Come on, Jenny, stop fooling with your makeup—we're late for the St. Valentine's Day party!"

Jenny's twin sister, Rose, was standing in the doorway. She wore a huge pink bow in her hair, and a long-sleeved blouse covered with bright red hearts.

"You're the vainest person I've ever met!" yelped Rose.

"Wait a minute," said Jenny. "I'm not looking at my makeup. I've got this lump on the right side of my cheek. . . ."

But Rose wasn't listening. This was the biggest dance of the year at Valley Pines High School, located in a Dallas, Texas, suburb, and the two 17-year-old seniors had been looking forward to it for months.

But now Jenny Kramer seemed distracted, uneasy, as Rose piloted the family's green-painted Chevy Vega toward the Valley Pines gym. She kept feeling her right cheek. Was she imaging that lump? No . . . there it was again—each time she pushed against the soft tissue flesh there, she could feel a mass of hard, unyielding tissue lurking beneath. Was it growing? My God, could it be a tumor?

She looked up. Rose was pulling the Vega into a parking space.

"What's the matter with you, Sad Sack?" cried Rose, as they exited the car and headed for the entrance of the gymnasium, where pink and scarlet streamers beckoned invitingly. "Come on, Jenny—be my Valentine!"

She hugged her sister hard. But Jenny kept on frowning, kept on probing the sore spot with the fingers of her right hand. They had reached the big double-doors of the gym, by now; already they could hear the loudspeakers booming inside:

*Whenever I'm near you,
It's like A HEAT WAVE. . .*

Then they were inside the huge, echoing gym, and looking for a coat-rack.

I'll have to tell Mom about it in the morning, Jenny kept reminding herself. . .

Three days later, she was sitting in the examining room of a Dallas Ear, Nose, and Throat (ENT) specialist, Dr. Harris Edgerton. Her worried mom, Connie Kramer, sat beside her.

"You've got what we call a 'hypertrophied lymph node'," Dr. Edgerton was saying, as he flipped the switch on an overhead slide projector.

Then, as the lights dimmed in the examining room and the screen lit up on the wall beside them, he continued, "Do you see the outline of the lymph node system, as I've marked it here? See how it runs down the cheek to the neck, then to the armpit? It's like knots along a string—with each one of the little nodes consisting of millions of special cells, macrophages, that fight disease and absorb foreign substances, or dead skin. . . "

The two of them, mother and daughter, were staring uncertainly at the screen.

"What we do," said Dr. Edgerton, "is to go in and take a tiny slice of tissue and look at it under the microscope. And if we don't like what we see, we simply remove the node. It's a harmless operation, really. Even if the cells in there should turn out to be cancerous, which isn't likely, we've probably caught the thing in time to eliminate any spread of the tumor."

Mrs. Kramer gasped, and reached for her big green pocketbook. "Did you say tumor?"

"It's possible, Mrs. Kramer. But not very likely—something on the order of one chance in a hundred."

But Mrs. Kramer, a thin, nervous-looking woman with hazel eyes, didn't seem very convinced. She was hugging the pocketbook in her lap, and rocking back and forth in her chair. "Take it out!" she suddenly cried to the startled doctor. "Just get rid of the damn thing!"

Jenny grabbed her momma's hand. "Calm down, Mother. It's a minor operation—local anesthetic!"

"I'm sure everything will be fine."

But it wasn't. On the day of the surgery, February 24, 1995, the Dallas ENT specialist failed miserably in his first and fundamental responsibility to his patient: above all, do no harm!

For reasons that remain unclear to this day, Dr. Edgerton chose to remove the swollen node, even though his biopsy indicated clearly that the hypertrophy of the tiny organ hadn't been triggered by a malignancy.

Had he simply been too eager to soothe the irrational fears of the patient's frightened mother and "take it out—get rid of the damn thing"?

Who knows? But the decision to remove the node wasn't actually the most critical mistake Dr. Edgerton made, in this classic case of surgical malpractice. In fact, the miscue that would haunt Jenny Kramer for the rest of her days occurred not at the site of the hypertrophied node, but a few millimeters away, at the junction of several important facial nerves.

Did the scalpel slip? Or did the harried Dr. Edgerton—who would see twelve different patients that day, along with performing this surgery, according to later testimony—simply lose his grip on the basics of human anatomy for a few crucial seconds?

Whatever the cause, the unhappy outcome was that Dr. Edgerton sliced through the major nerve-cluster. Recognizing his mistake within a few seconds, he hurriedly attempted to place a graft on the affected tissue—in a longshot bid to reconnect the severed nerves. But as usually happens in such cases, the graft was rejected and the nerve-damage became permanent.

And the results were unfortunate, to say the least.

Even though Jenny Kramer's harmlessly swollen lymph node was benign, requiring no surgery whatsoever, she had been compelled to endure a facial operation—and an operation which left the entire right side of her face permanently "drooping" and completely paralyzed!

In Jenny's unhappy case, the disfigurement would prove to be quite significant. Always fretful about her appearance, the high school senior was devastated by the "droopy look" that the paralysis gave to her features. So upsetting was the impact on her adolescent psyche, in fact, that within two years of graduating from Valley Pines, she developed a serious drinking problem that soon deepened into full-blown, life-threatening alcoholism.

Truth, Lies and the OR

It took Jenny Kramer more than six years—and about $50,000 in psychiatrists' fees—to unsnarl the psychological tangle that had been triggered by Dr. Edgerton's careless surgery.

A ghastly medical mistake! Believe it or not, however, a Texas jury later found the Dallas ENT specialist innocent of malpractice, while rejecting Jenny Kramer's bid to collect reimbursement for the tens of thousands of dollars that her family had spent on medical and related costs, as a result of the botched surgery!

While no one should attempt to "read the mind" of a jury (an impossible assignment, anyway, as I discovered long ago!), it seems likely that in this case the jurors were so swayed by the word "cancer" that they voted to find the pathetic Dr. Edgerton innocent of negligence.

Were they correct? Of course not. The facts in this sad case clearly demonstrate the overwhelming incompetence of the doctor. Ask yourself: is there a surgeon on Planet Earth who can't tell you the location of the facial nerve? Make no mistake: the "standards of ordinary care" were violated here; a more careful dissection of the node would have saved the young lady from a lifetime of emotional pain brought on by the disfigurement.

But the jury in *Kramer v. Edgerton and Hillcrest Hospital* obviously didn't agree with this assessment; as happens all too frequently in malpractice litigation in this country, they seemed to be swayed by the laymen's tendency to protect the doctor at all costs.

****

Rx: The Toughest Challenge in Winning a Malpractice Case is Convincing the Jury to Reject Medical Misinformation.

During many years of serving as an expert witness in litigation involving negligent doctors, I've seen many medical malpractice cases that should have been won, but weren't.

F. W. Ernst, M.D. — William G. Pace III, M. D.

I think it might be useful to share a few of those losing court battles with you, in the hope of making clear just how judges and attorneys manage the complicated business of adjudicating malpractice in this country of ours. Rest assured, however: I'm not really interested in attacking the medical community in this "inside look" at the world of medical malpractice—not at all. Rather, I'm simply hoping to provide information to patients and health-care consumers that will help them make better choices about both health-care and legal issues.

With that said, let me begin by describing one of the major areas of malpractice to which I've been summoned time and time again, as an expert witness: cases involving injury to the spinal accessory nerve caused by a poorly executed posterior cervical lymph node biopsy.

Interestingly enough, I was recently chastised by a surgical colleague, a neurosurgeon, for testifying that this accident usually occurs as the result of negligence. But I must stand by my assessment: I don't think there's any question but that such a loss to the patient clearly lies outside the proper standards of care.

In the first place, remember that the posterior cervical lymph nodes are rarely, if ever, involved in malignancy. As a matter of fact, the only time I've ever seen them enlarged was during attacks of "cat scratch fever" or perhaps during measles. (Neither condition justifies a biopsy, however.)

But if surgery should be mandated for some reason, the surgeon should certainly remain aware of the fact that the spinal accessory nerve is positioned close to that area, and must be first located and then protected at all costs. Why? It's simple: the injuries that I've seen inflicted when negligence occurs in this procedure are simply devastating; quite frequently, the patients end up not only with "winging of the scapula," but also with persistent pain, discomfort and dysfunction of the shoulder girdle.

Truth, Lies and the OR

I suppose the lesson for the patient who finds a lump on the back of his or her neck below the ear (in what we call the posterior cervical triangle) is this: you must be certain to obtain more than one medical opinion about the advisability of biopsying such a mass.

If a biopsy does seem called for, the patient should select either a plastic surgeon or perhaps even a neurosurgeon and then discuss the procedure in detail with him or her before the operation, along with the potential for injury to the spinal accessory nerve.

You should ask these specialists a crucial question: Is the surgery absolutely required?

Remember that the odds of the tissue being malignant are about one in a thousand. Still, your discussion with the medical personnel should touch on the recommended course of action, if a section of the nerve is found to be malignant—along with the potential for a simultaneous graft, if a segment of the nerve must be resected. At the very least, such a pre-operative discussion would make clear on the pathology section just what surgical steps are mandated, and just what steps will be taken to protect the vital nerve. (In this way, you can usually avoid the trauma of waking up after surgery to find your shoulder paralyzed.)

Another interesting case of surgical malpractice in which I was called upon to offer an opinion was a botched operation to correct carpal tunnel syndrome. In this dispute, the defendant surgeon stated that he had used a variation of his own on the procedure to correct the syndrome, which is caused when ligaments tighten across the bottom of the wrist, below the palm of the hand, resulting in numbness and dysfunction of the fingers, along with severe pain in the hand and fingers.

The standard treatment calls for cutting the transverse carpal ligament, which is a tough bunch of fibers that cross the palm from the base of the thumb to the base of the small finger, right at the crease of the wrist, at the bottom of the so-called "heartline" of the palm. The usual procedure for this problem requires an incision which extends up and into the palm and down onto the wrist, so that all the fibers of the ligament can be identified and cut, and the structures underneath it can be freed of pressure.

In more recent years, a newer, laparoscopic technique has been perfected to relieve carpal tunnel syndrome. This technique is less invasive with a much quicker recovery period. In fact, many patients may be able to return to work within several days following surgery. This technique is not without possible injury to the median nerve when done by an inexperienced surgeon. Be sure you choose a surgeon who has considerable training and experience in this technique to help ensure positive results. Do not hesitate to ask about a surgeon's credentials before allowing him or her to operate on you using this technique.

The patient in this case did not improve, however, and later sought help elsewhere at a special clinic where the operation was accomplished properly. And the second surgeon didn't hesitate to criticize the first, while describing his colleague's earlier dissection as "the smallest incision that I've ever seen." He also noted that none of the fibers of the ligament had been cut during the first surgery.

This fact, alone, would appear to offer prima facie evidence for a case in which "res ipsa loquitur" ("the thing speaks for itself"). Since it was quite evident, during the second operation, that none of the fibers had been cut earlier, there could be no denying that the first surgery (for which the patient had been billed) had simply not taken place!

This incident amounted to little more than sham surgery. And yet the jury in this case somehow concluded that the surgeon had performed the services required of him, and found no evidence of deviation from standards of care.

I beg to differ, however.

Truth, Lies and the OR

In my opinion, if a patient discusses a certain operation with a surgeon, and then the surgeon proceeds to make an incision in the skin, but doesn't complete the operation for which he has contracted, that's a deviation from the standard of care. Apparently, though, the jury applied the principle of "let the buyer beware" en route to dismissing the plaintiff's claims.

Surely, this patient would have been well advised to seek out the services of a competent hand clinic, after learning the diagnosis. He should not have simply depended on the services of the local surgeon, who, as it turned out, performed every type of surgery in the book, and had no special training of any kind in hand surgery.

In an earlier chapter, we discussed the importance of making sure that the surgeon who will operate on you is an expert in that particular surgical specialty. To have allowed a general surgeon—who rarely if ever works on carpal ligaments—to operate on your carpal tunnel syndrome makes about as much sense as allowing a general practitioner to remove a brain tumor because he had once done a craniotomy in medical school, as a fifth assistant in the operating room!

Still, the patient deserved better than the jury's flawed verdict in this poorly decided case.

One of the most incredible miscarriages of justice I've encountered during a jury trial occurred in Tennessee a few years ago. In that case, I was consulted about a patient who had been operated on for a problem of morbid obesity. The surgeon had never really worked on a case like this ... and in the course of the operation, he removed the spleen because of an injury to it during the surgery that he couldn't control.

Although the loss of the spleen clearly involved some slippage from standards of care, it didn't necessarily involve outright negligence. And yet the incident did require dedicated follow-up on the part of the surgeon and the hospital medical team.

Unfortunately for our patient in this case, however, the surgeon chose to go on a small vacation soon after the spleen removal, while turning the care of the patient over to a colleague who had never seen—or done—any of these procedures, and who was supposed to be responsible for the immediate post-operative care.

Now, one of the problems that frequently crops up in the post-operative course of treatment after a splenectomy is the danger of pancreatitis, or injury to the pancreas.

In this case, that problem did emerge, and the patient was discovered, soon after the surgery, to be running a very high amylase count that required immediate and aggressive medical attention.

Sadly, however, no such treatment was afforded the patient throughout the first post-operative night. By morning, as a result, the patient was suffering from falling blood pressure, declining urinary output, and a rising pulse—all indications that he was drifting into shock with pancreatitis, as part of a potentially fatal disorder that had been entirely preventable.

Soon it was apparent that the patient was sliding into deep shock and would require immediate aggressive therapy, including replacement of fluids and colloids, if his life were to be saved.

Once again, however, the patient languished without treatment. And when the nurses attempted to get him out of bed, a few hours later, his eyes rolled back and he appeared faint. The nurses responded by snapping an ampule of ammonia under his nose—to which the patient reacted by falling to the floor, where he was pronounced dead after a failure to resuscitate him.

Once again, the facts in this hideous example of malpractice would appear to speak for themselves. This was clear-cut negligence, a monstrosity of medical care in which the raging pancreatitis was allowed to progress, untreated up to and past the point of death.

There was simply no justification for what happened to this patient, and during the autopsy it was noted that he was also suffering from acute tubular necrosis of the kidneys—a condition which occurs prior to death, and which can be diagnosed only by microscopic examination of the kidneys after death. Acute tubular necrosis is a situation in which the kidney tissue dies as the result of low blood pressure, or so-called "shock." The patient had clearly exhibited the symptoms of shock before his death, yet the lawyers for the defense continued to insist that this fact could only have been demonstrated during a post-mortem exam.

The reason behind the defense's refusal to admit that the patient had been suffering from shock before his demise became clear a few days later in the trial when a Fellow of the American College of Surgeons testified under oath that the patient had died from "acute ammonia intoxication" as a result of the nurse snapping the ampule under his nose. In other words, said the defense expert with a straight face, the patient hadn't died from shock and pancreatitis. No way. Instead, he'd been killed by a whiff of ammonia under his nose!

It sounds ludicrous, but this particular trial soon became a classic case of the difficulty that's frequently involved in educating the jury to the facts in medical malpractice.

Day after day, we did our best to explain the physiology and pharmacology of pancreatitis, while trying to fend off the local Tennessee experts who were insisting that the patient had died of ammonia intoxication and that pancreatitis simply hadn't been a factor.

Of course, the idea that an ammonia ampule could trigger "instant death" seems laughable on reflection, and yet this jury appeared to accept it—probably because the bizarre theory was being advanced by one of their own doctors.

F. W. Ernst, M.D. — William G. Pace III, M. D.

In my view, this case was a classic instance of a jury's failure to render a just verdict... a fact which meant that the destitute family of this victim of malpractice would go uncompensated.

It was a travesty, no doubt about it. And yet it's clear that if we keep asking juries to make these crucial medical judgments—while being fed misinformation by the defense—then we're going to be faced with occasional miscarriages of the kind that produced this pathetic verdict.

I suppose the lesson for the plaintiff in any malpractice suit is this: no matter how airtight and perfect you think your case is, you can be certain that if it comes before a jury, it will be judged in an entirely different light—after the defense has presented its version of events and its expert witnesses have testified.

Another memorable case in which I was involved centered on the dialysis of a little girl in a small South Carolina town. She had developed Dupuytren's contracture, and the local vascular surgeon was the attending physician. Interestingly, he'd previously written a medical article for publication which described a cephalic vein shunt.

He pointed out in his article, specifically, that these shunts should not be used for a minimum of six weeks after they've been created, because they must grow tight to the skin to prevent development of any large blood clot in the soft tissue, and they need time to heal properly.

The operation on the young girl was performed in order to provide a chronic shunt to facilitate her dialysis for terminal kidney disease. On the third day after the shunt was installed, there was a consultation between the nephrologist (kidney doctor) and the vascular surgeon, in which they discussed using that shunt immediately, since they needed an access site.

Strangely, the vascular surgeon decided to violate all of his own rules, and agreed that they could go ahead and use the shunt. And the results were disastrous: at ten o'clock the next morning, during dialysis, a huge hematoma (blood clot) developed, precisely where the doctor had predicted it would happen.

The nurses in the dialysis unit attempted in vain several times to locate either of the two doctors, but were unable to do so. They elevated the patient's arm, placed ice bags on it, and applied some degree of pressure, but continued the dialysis.

After nearly an hour, they managed to reach the nephrologist on the phone. Instead of visiting the patient, however, he merely prescribed a continuation of the ice bags and more dialysis. This was accomplished, but, at the completion of the dialysis, the nurses noted that this was the largest blood clot they'd ever seen, and also that the patient was screaming in pain.

Repeated efforts to contact the doctor failed, and there was never a call back. In fact, no physician actually saw the patient until ten o'clock the following morning, nearly 24 hours after the injury. At that time, the physician's notes indicated that she would certainly require decompression of the arm—and that since it couldn't be done under local anesthesia, a general anesthetic would be required.

Before that step could be taken, however, the patient had to be dialyzed again, and so nothing was done for another 24 hours, until the nurses noted that the patient was having trouble moving her fingers and was still screaming in pain.

At last the patient was taken to surgery, where, under general anesthesia, the area was opened up, and—precisely as the surgeon had predicted—an examination showed that the needle had passed through the front and out the back of the vein, causing the enormous blood clot that had compressed the upper arm.

Of course, it was a very simple matter to suture closed these two holes on either side of the vein and evacuate the blood from the upper arm, removing the pressure from the lower arm.

F. W. Ernst, M.D. — William G. Pace III, M. D.

By the time this was accomplished, however, the chronic pressure had caused what is known as a Dupuytren's type syndrome, in which the compression of the nerves of the forearm results in a claw-like hand, which contracts into a little fist which is essentially worthless for the rest of the patient's life.

Clearly, the doctor's procrastination and failure to act in an obvious emergency were the causes of this little girl's injury.

Unfortunately for this patient however, the jury returned a verdict in favor of the surgeon, with the following admonition to the plaintiff's lawyer: "Son, we simply don't lose malpractice cases here in this state!"

Perhaps the lesson here is that patients and their families simply have to insist on their due process rights prior to development of an injury, not afterwards.

In addition, a surgical patient should always be certain that the surgeon on his or her case in a specialty area, such as vascular access for dialysis, is thoroughly competent and aware of the factors involved, and that he or she has performed many of these procedures, not simply a few of them.

In another unusual case, one of the attorneys with whom I've had a wonderful working relationship over the years first consulted me back in 1990 about a patient with a broken femur. As often happens in this situation (since the defense attorneys aren't spending their own money), the doctor's lawyers will proceed through a deposition simply in order to determine if the expert for the plaintiff is believable—or if, indeed, he can be impeached and discredited.

In the broken femur case that was presented to me, a patient had a fainting spell in a restaurant. The physician at the hospital to which he was taken concluded that he'd had a small stroke. The patient was subsequently sedated and put into a bed without side rails—a negligent act in any hospital.

Since the patient was neither restrained nor supervised, he naturally tried to climb out of bed, fell and was found on the floor. He was then taken to the X-ray department—where his films were promptly misread. The fracture was one in which the head of the femur was impacted on the femoral neck—a fairly common situation—but one in which it is possible for the X-ray to give the appearance of a normal femoral bone.

But if such a fracture has actually occurred, you can be sure that it will simply fall apart if untreated, as this one did. A few days later, in fact, the patient's fracture disintegrated and he toppled to the floor. He was then discovered to have a disimpacted fracture of the femoral neck.

Ordinarily, of course, this type of case should be settled without any questions and without wasting the insurance company's money on depositions. I wrote a letter that was designed to serve as the basis for such a settlement, but the matter was nonetheless carried forward through an expensive and wasteful deposition before the defendants finally did decide to settle in favor of the plaintiff.

This case provides a very clear lesson for any client whose family member might be admitted under circumstances in which he or she might not be mentally capable: make sure there is adequate nursing coverage and/or restraints for the patient, and supervision during the course of the hospital stay.

If, under any circumstances, a relative should fall out of bed, assume the absolute worst until you see proof-positive that the worst didn't happen! Remember that the simple reading of an X-ray that shows there's no fracture is no assurance whatsoever that one hasn't occurred. Remember, also, that a sub-capital fracture with impaction can be misread very easily by an X-ray department.

The unhappy outcome of this case was that the patient died—when the simple insertion of a nail at the time of the initial injury could have prevented the entire scenario. The lesson for the attending doctor should be equally important: if a patient who is mentally or physically impaired doesn't get good supervision, a disaster looms on the horizon! And if it does happen that such a patient falls from bed, you must obtain more than superficial assurance that no injury occurred.

These cases all show us the necessity of becoming an informed medical patient or family member. You simply can't wait until after a mistake has been made to begin asking questions!

It's true that jury verdicts are often unfair. But make no mistake: even a successful jury award can't make up for injuries—or even death—suffered by those we love. **As a patient, your best defense is knowledge—be informed!**

IN SUMMARY

- Surgical patients and other health-care consumers can protect themselves against medical negligence quite effectively by taking the trouble to understand why so many malpractice cases end in defeat for the plaintiffs—even though the complaining patients were, indeed, injured by incompetent physicians.

- Surgical patients should be sure to obtain a second and even a third opinion before agreeing to have a tissue mass biopsy if it impinges on a nerve. If such procedures are flawed, they can produce permanent paralysis.

- One of the great difficulties in obtaining justice before small town juries in medical malpractice cases is that they will frequently do their best to "protect" the local doctor regardless of the facts in the case.

- Even if you win a substantial malpractice award, it can't make up for injury to a loved one.

**REMEMBER: as a patient, knowledge is your best defense.
Be forewarned!**

F. W. Ernst, M.D. — William G. Pace III, M. D.

EPILOGUE

Open, honest, and stress-free communication between patient and physician is of critical importance in establishing a healthy, working relationship between these two parties. Furthermore, this type of communication is equally important for the complete transfer of important medical information between these two parties so the patient can receive optimum care for his/her medical needs. According to one report, appointments in doctors' offices last an average of 15 minutes. If you are fortunate, you convey your basic medical complaints and get the majority of your questions answered in easily understood language in this time period. However, even the most pro-active, informed medical consumer can leave a doctor's office still unsure about critical information regarding his/her diagnosis or treatment.

Here are some suggestions to help make your visit to your doctor more productive and decrease chances of communication breakdowns.

1. **Be a list maker**. Although this suggestion may seem trite, it really does help to ensure more complete communication with your doctor. Take unhurried time before your appointment to list all the topics or items you want to cover with your doctor. Be sure you include your symptoms, how long you have had them, and any other information you may recall. **Remember:** what you may think is an insignificant fact may be very important information to your doctor. After making your list, go through it again and prioritize it. This will help ensure that your most important topics get discussed.
2. **Set an agenda. (Why are you there?)** At the start of your appointment, verbalize to your doctor how you wish the time to be spent. If you don't clarify up-front what you hope to

achieve in this visit, important points may not get covered. Ask your doctor if he agrees with this agenda. If you are clear in your wishes and your doctor seems to ignore you or put you down, then this should be a clear warning sign that you are in the wrong office. Get out of there, and go to a doctor who will communicate with you!

3. **Be direct**. Do not be intimidated by any doctor or allow any doctor to intimidate you in the communication process. We are not "gods on pedestals." Don't put us there. Be very open, specific, and honest in your communication.

4. **Ask questions about a referral**. If your doctor is going to refer you to a specialist, ask about his/her credentials and what you should do to prepare for your visit to that specialist. Unfortunately, specialists get advance information from the referring doctor less than 30% of the time. So, take your list to the specialist and be prepared to discuss your problem.

5. **Don't tie up your doctor's time with information**. Many patients today are researching their medical conditions on the Internet or in other sources. This is an important part of becoming a knowledgeable, pro-active patient. However, don't hand your doctor pages of printed or written material during your appointment. Summarize in less than one page any information you feel is important that you wish to discuss.

6. **Verbalize reasons behind your requests**. Perhaps you have a specific test or tests you wish to have done and your doctor denies that request. Explain to the doctor why you are asking for those tests. In this way, you may either persuade your doctor to do the test, or better understand why he/she won't.

7. **Voice your complaints**. Give your doctor honest feedback. Don't complain behind his/her back. If you feel intimidated

about confronting a doctor on a matter that distresses you, write him/her a note and explain fully your complaint. Give your doctor a chance to make things right. If your doctor is still unresponsive, consider a letter to the physician's practice group. If a physician or his/her group continues to be unresponsive to your complaint, find another doctor.

8. **Clearly identify the cause of any disagreement**. If you and your doctor don't agree on a diagnosis, examination results, or treatment plan, take a few steps back and discuss what is at the bottom of your disagreement. Do you think something was missed or ignored? Have an honest discussion with your doctor about how to resolve these differences.

9. **Summarize your visit**. Take time to review any tests ordered, medications prescribed, or suggested lifestyles changes to which you have agreed. This approach can go a long way to preventing any misunderstandings.

F. W. Ernst, M.D. — William G. Pace III, M. D.

AFTERWORD

It happens to every author, somewhere near the completion of a major book.

Suddenly, you find yourself staring out the window, while asking the same question over and over again, "Have I accomplished the goals I set out in the beginning?"

With your permission, I'd like to share a few of the thoughts that have emerged from such "philosophical moments" after working on this volume for a year.

A piece of wisdom one of my outstanding teachers, Dr. C. Ronald Stephen, passed on to me many years ago was, "Don't be one of the first to grab onto a new drug or technique. Rather, be advised, wait until it has established a track record and see where it levels off. Then decide if this new drug or technique should be incorporated into your practice." As patient consumers, we—yes, we as physicians may be patients, too—might avoid many potential problems if we did not subject our bodies to something "new" or "in vogue" but rather waited until the track record had been established.

We pay a premium price when a new drug or technique first becomes available. With time, this price will generally decrease. Some patients take an alternative path by going to a country to receive drugs and/or treatment which is unavailable in the United States. All too often, there are large amounts of money spent on travel and treatment without benefits of the hoped for healing.

Is there a single message we have tried to convey in **Truth, Lies, and the O.R.**? Actually, I hope not: for my co-author and I have done our best to appeal to a broad spectrum of readers, and to the wide variety of questions that such an audience might have. But one theme does emerge on page after page: as strong patient advocates, both Dr. Pace and I hope that this book will increase patients' awareness about potential medical pitfalls and problems that can be avoided by choosing health-care providers more wisely—and by seeking out the best treatment alternatives in any given situation. By being better informed patients, we can engage in clear dialogue with medical professionals and make reasonable requests.

We hope our medical colleagues will read this book with open minds. Furthermore, we hope you will realize that our endeavor is constructive, an honest look at some of the problems in our medical profession and an attempt to find solutions. If you treat your patients properly—as you would wish to be treated in their shoes—malpractice problems often evaporate before they ever materialize.

It's time for physicians everywhere to understand one basic fact: many of today's malpractice lawsuits are taking place because the "art" of medicine has been increasingly ignored in recent years. The compassionate, empathetic side of our practice has been on the decline, while the "science" of medicine, the "high-tech" application of machines and instruments to what are, after all, human beings, has been soaring off the charts. In a word, we've been paying too much attention to the physical bodies of our patients in recent years, and too little attention to their hearts and minds.

When you stop going to see patients in the hospital but still send them a bill, when you are abrupt with a patient who wants an extra five minutes, dismissing him or her because there are others in the waiting room, when you won't attend to their emotional needs or cares, when surgeries are canceled or postponed because YOU have allowed your office staff to double-book you . . . these are causes for many lawsuits. They are not demonstrable forms of negligence and really are reasons for lawsuits that should not happen.

Every medical professional surely understands that quality "one-on-one" sharing between doctor and patient can facilitate healing. (And that's especially true, if you accept the estimate of experts who say that more than 50 percent of human illnesses are emotionally triggered!) So the question becomes: given the present trends in medical treatment and philosophy in this country, how can we improve quality of care and thus improve the "art" of medicine? **I wish I had the answer.**

How do you reason, for example, with large "for-profit" corporations on the stock market, whose only concern is the "bottom line"? They profess that quality patient care is a top priority, BUT, when a physician chooses a new drug or technique to treat a medical condition, and it is more expensive than an older, less effective alternative, management may balk: "Doctor, you are cutting into our profits too much!"

The Health Maintenance Organizations (HMOs) are creating problems for us all. With the emphasis on primary care physicians and a decreased use of trained specialists, I hear about increasing numbers of patients being misdiagnosed. Furthermore, by the time they are finally sent to a specialist, it may be too late to effect a cure. Meanwhile, the HMO's continue to rack up **huge profits**.

It is impossible for any physician to master all of the knowledge in general medicine today. And yet, that's precisely what the "HMO concept" requires! By making the primary care physician the "gatekeeper," the HMO limits access to specialists. Furthermore, when the gatekeeper is rewarded with a salary bonus for coming in under budget on patient costs—and if he's punished for budget overruns—how willing do you think he or she will be to refer patients to specialists for vitally needed treatment?

It's a medical shame. And it's also the kind of medical issue that this book directly addresses. In an attempt to help patients avoid some of the problems and pitfalls in medical care, we've done our best to emphasize the importance of patients informing themselves about their medical conditions and their treatment alternatives.

F. W. Ernst, M.D. — William G. Pace III, M. D.

When it comes to evaluating a surgeon's ability in the operating room, the anesthesia personnel and the other professionals in the OR are your best source of knowledge. They are really the only source—since they are the only staff who can observe, up close, just how well a surgeon manages difficult and stressful situations during a procedure. If you know someone in one of these professions, that person may be your best friend in helping you decide on your choice of surgeons.

We also hope you'll use this book. After spending a year or so struggling to get the right words on the page, it's our sincere wish that **Truth, Lies and the O.R.** will serve you—and thousands of medical consumers like you—for many, many years to come!

ABOUT THE AUTHORS

FREDERICK W. ERNST, M.D.

Dr. Ernst is a practicing anesthesiologist for over 40 years with sub-specialties in pediatric and outpatient anesthesia. Prior to semi-retiring, he was medical director of two outpatient surgery centers in Alabama. He has authored 11 scientific publications and delivered over 60 presentations at national professional meetings. For six years, his syndicated medical-consumer newspaper column, "America's Ralph Nader of Medicine Speaks Out," was carried in over 70 newspapers nationwide. Presently, he does patients' rights advocacy work, private consulting, and medical-legal expert witness testimony for both plaintiff and defense counsel in medical malpractice cases.

WILLIAM G. PACE III, M.D.

Dr. Pace was Professor of Surgery and Assistant Dean for the Ohio State University College of Medicine from 1959-1991. From 1991 until his death, he held the title of Professor Emeritus. He authored well over 100 scientific publications, served as a contributing editor for three surgical textbooks, and produced 17 scientific movies. During the last 25 years of his life, he was in great demand as an expert witness in numerous medical malpractice cases.

F. W. Ernst, M.D. — William G. Pace III, M. D.

NANCY G. SPEAR, Ph.D., CRNA

A graduate of Mercy Hospital School of Anesthesia, Pittsburgh, Pennsylvania, Dr. Spear received her doctorate in education, communications, and technology from the University of Pittsburgh and is the former director of the Western Penn Hospital School of Nurse Anesthesia in Pittsburgh. Currently, she is employed as a locum tenens anesthetist and serves on the editorial board of Current Reviews for Nurse Anesthetists. When not in the hospital surgical suite, she can be found pursuing her second career as a professional photographer.

ABOUT THE EDITORS

DINAH BLANKENSHIP

An English teacher for 25 years, Ms. Blankenship was chairwoman of the Department of English, Dothan High School. Dothan, Alabama. During her career, she conducted numerous professional workshops on topics of English and was listed in Who's Who Among High School Teachers. Now retired, she devotes time to her passion, genealogy, and serves as the Current Regent for the Daughters of the American Revolution.

TOM NUGENT

Science Journalist, Tom Nugent is the author of several books on medicine and health in the workplace, including **Breakthroughs in American Medicine** (Detroit Medical Center Press) and **Death at Buffalo Creek** (W. W. Norton). Nugent is a National Endowment for the Humanities Fellow in Journalism, and was awarded a Fund for Constitutional Government grant to investigate the environmental effects of strip mining for coal in Appalachia. Nominated by the Baltimore Sun for the Pulitzer Prize in 1980, Nugent has also written for the Chicago Tribune, the Washington Post, the Boston Globe, the University of Chicago Magazine and many other publications in recent years and often writes about medicine and health.

F. W. Ernst, M.D. — William G. Pace III, M. D.

GLOSSARY

ABMS (American Board of Medical Specialists): oversees the administration of the 24 specialty boards in the U.S.

Ambulatory Care Center: an outpatient treatment center. With reference to surgery, this would be a care unit where patients have their surgery and go home the same day.

Anesthesiologist (MDA): the medical specialist who provides pain relief and keeps you asleep during surgery.

ASA (American Society of Anesthesiologists): the professional organization for anesthesiologists.

BIS (bi-spectral index): the clinical monitor that records the brain activity of a patient under general anesthesia.

BMI (body mass index): a test that calculates the degree of obesity in a person.

Board certification: the highest attestation of competency a physician practicing in the U.S. can obtain. This certification is granted by one of the 24 boards of the ABMS following successful completion of an extensive examination process.

CRNA (Certified Registered Nurse Anesthetist): a registered nurse who has successfully completed training in anesthesia and then passes a national certifying examination.

EKG (electrocardiogram): an electronic tracing of the heart's electrical activity.

Fellowship training: specialty training beyond the basic residency training in any given area of a medical specialty.

G-I (gastrointestinal): refers to the entire digestive system of the body from the mouth to the rectum.

HMO (Health Maintenance Organization): a health-care provider organization in which selected physicians administer health care to participating members.

Hypovolemia: decreased circulating blood volume.

Intravenous (IV): the route by which drugs, fluids, or chemotherapy are administered into a patient's vein.

JCAHO (Joint Commission for Accreditation of Healthcare Organizations): one of several national organizations that accredit healthcare facilities—primarily hospitals and ambulatory surgery centers for this organization.

Matching Plan: the national organization that matches medical college graduates with residency training programs in the U.S.

Peritonitis: inflammation of the peritoneal lining, the membrane that lines the abdominal cavity.

Primary Care Physician: a non-medical specialist who provides basic medical care to patients (generally refers to a general practitioner or an internist).

Resection: a cutting off or cutting out of a particular part of the human body.

Spinal: anything that refers to the bony spine or the spinal cord.

Stomach stapling: making the stomach smaller through the use of surgical staples.

Suction lipectomy: the process of removing fat tissue from the body utilizing a suction machine.

Type II Diabetes: a group of varieties of diabetes that occur predominantly in adults. This type is generally considered to be non-insulin dependent.

Volume: the space occupied by a substance, usually a gas or a liquid.

F. W. Ernst, M.D. — William G. Pace III, M. D.

America's Ralph Nader of Medicine Speaks Out!

For speaking engagements or to schedule radio/TV interviews please contact Dr. F. W. Ernst at www.drfernst.com or go to www.warrenpublishing.net